Clare B. Unley M.D.

ARTHRITIS
IN BLACK AND WHITE

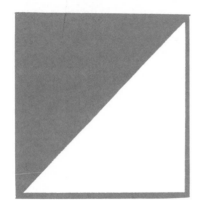

To: Claire,
You'll never see
Gout in the hospital
grove in this book,
You'll have to wait
for the gray zone.

Anne C. Brower

ANNE C. BROWER, M.D.

Formerly, Professor of Radiology and Orthopaedic
Surgery, Georgetown University Hospital,
Washington, D.C.

1988

W. B. SAUNDERS COMPANY
Harcourt Brace Jovanovich, Inc.
Philadelphia, London, Toronto, Montreal, Sydney, Tokyo

W. B. SAUNDERS COMPANY
Harcourt Brace Jovanovich, Inc.

West Washington Square
Philadelphia, PA 19105

Library of Congress Cataloging-in-Publication Data

Brower, Anne C.

Arthritis in black and white.

1. Arthritis—Diagnosis.   2. Diagnosis, Radioscopic.
   I. Title.   [DNLM: 1. Arthritis—radiography.
   WE 344 B877a]

RC933.B76   1988   616.7'22'0757   87–20758

ISBN 0–7216–2243–7

Production Manager: Frank Polizzano

Manuscript Editor: Donna Walker

Illustration Coordinator: Kenneth Green

Indexer: Donna Walker

Arthritis in Black and White   ISBN   0–7216–2243–7

Last digit is the print number: 9   8   7   6   5   4   3   2   1

to
D.O.W.

ACKNOWLEDGMENTS

This book, although a long-time dream, is now a reality because of the tremendous efforts of the many people I am deeply indebted to:

KAREN KELLOUGH—from her consistently accurate preparation of the manuscript.

ROBERT IRVING—for his excellent photography of all the radiographs.

ANN BIGNELL—for her clear illustrations.

ALL MY RESIDENTS—for their inspiration.

DON RESNICK—for his encouragement.

LARRY ELLIOTT—for his provision of time.

MY MOTHER—for her understanding and support.

W. B. SAUNDERS—most especially Donna Walker, Frank Polizzano, and Lorraine Kilmer, for the final product.

PREFACE

This book is the result of requests from many residents who have heard my simplistic approach to the radiographic diagnosis of arthritic disease. All of the material in the book has been printed in some form in other books, as well as in multiple journal articles. The purpose of this work is to provide a small, practical book organized so as to allow relative ease in accurate diagnosis of arthritic disease through the radiograph. It is designed for practicing general radiologists, family practitioners, internists, and rheumatologists to use in day-to-day practice.

It is entitled *Arthritis in Black and White* to indicate that (1) it deals with arthritis as seen on the radiograph, and (2) it is a very basic, simple book illustrating the hallmarks of the more common arthropathies. It is not meant to be an extensive reference book; it does not illustrate all of the radiographic aspects of arthritic disease. It illustrates only the hallmarks of the arthropathies, not the deviations or "gray zones" of the various arthropathies.

The radiographic diagnosis of arthritic disease depends upon the excellence and appropriateness of the image obtained, as discussed in the first chapter of this book. The role of all imaging modalities is presented. Today, however, the plain film radiograph remains the imaging modality of choice. Therefore, the focus of this book centers on plain film interpretation.

The book is designed to be used easily and quickly in approaching any radiograph obtained on unknown arthritic disease. For the reader's convenience the book is divided into two sections. The first section illustrates an approach to analyzing the radiographic changes in a specific joint and the common arthropathies that produce those changes in that particular joint. The second section illustrates the radiographic hallmarks of each of the common arthropathies. Thus the book might be used in the following way: When analyzing the radiograph of a knee on which the referring physician has questioned the possibility of rheumatoid arthritis, the user may turn to the chapter on rheumatoid arthritis in Section II and observe the hallmarks of rheumatoid arthritis as it presents in the knee. If the problem radiograph does not fit the hallmarks of rheumatoid arthritis, the user may then turn to the chapter on the knee in Section I and through the approach described arrive at the appropriate diagnosis.

The radiographic diagnosis of arthritic disease is a difficult subject. I can only hope that this book will provide an easy starting place for the interested physician. However, I am reminded of a paragraph written by F. Spilsbury in 1774:

> The disorder termed the Gout is difficult to cure, and occasions exquisite pain and uneasiness to the patient, and trouble and perplexity to the physician to discover the nature, cause and a remedy for this excruciating malady; books upon books have been wrote in different ages by men of ingenuity and learning, and much practice without the desired amendation, as might reasonably be hoped for from their abilities and experience; that I am almost disheartened from throwing in my mite, did not the desire of relieving preponderate, therefore shall give my thoughts on the subject, crude and barren as they are.

ANNE C. BROWER

CONTENTS

chapter 1

IMAGING TECHNIQUES AND MODALITIES

Evaluation of any articular disorder involves imaging the affected joints with the most appropriate modality. Imaging documents not only the extent and severity of joint involvement, but also the progression or regression of disease. More importantly, in the patient who presents with vague, complex, or confusing clinical symptoms, imaging often allows a specific diagnosis to be made. The modalities available for imaging are conventional radiography, conventional tomography, computed tomography, bone scintigraphy, ultrasonography, and magnetic resonance imaging. The role that each of these modalities may play in the evaluation of the patient with articular disease is discussed.

CONVENTIONAL RADIOGRAPHY

Evaluation of articular disease should begin with the conventional radiograph, which is the best modality to evaluate accurately any subtle change occurring in the bone. If high-quality radiographs are obtained in properly positioned patients, accurate evaluation can often be made without further studies.

A high-quality study demands that a high-resolution, fine-detail imaging system be used, especially on the extremities, to detect subtle disease. There are numerous film/screen combinations available, and the system utilized depends upon the individual radiography department. Generally, the lower the system speed, the higher the resolution. Today most departments employ a single screen/film combination with system speeds of 80 to 100 for this necessary resolution.

The symptomatic joint should be imaged in appropriate positions. It should be radiographed in at least two different projections. While one view may appear entirely normal, a second view taken at a 90-degree angle to the first view often shows significant abnormality (Fig. 1–1). Special views are available and should be utilized when imaging specific joints for articular diseases. The important positions for several of the joints commonly imaged are discussed below.

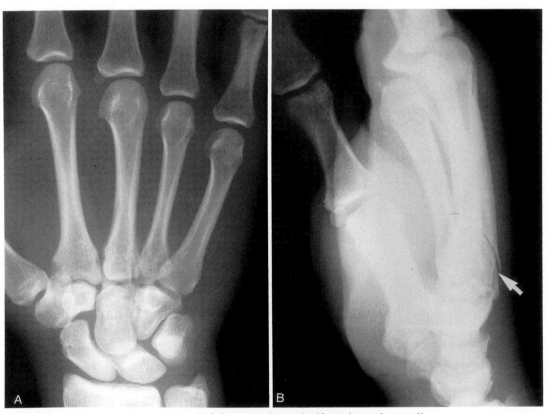

FIGURE 1–1. *A*, PA view of the metacarpals fails to reveal any significant bony abnormality. *B*, Lateral view of the same hand (taken 90 degrees to the PA view) shows a fracture through the proximal end of the shaft of the 3rd metacarpal (arrow).

1. Hand and Wrist

The posteroanterior (PA) and Norgaard views of the hands and wrists provide the most information if only two views are to be obtained. The PA view gives information on mineralization and soft tissue changes. The Norgaard view is used to demonstrate early erosive disease. The Norgaard view is an AP oblique view, or the oblique view opposite that routinely obtained. It has been described as the "You're in good hands with All-state" or "ball-catcher's" view. It profiles the radial aspect of the base of the proximal phalanges in the hand and the triquetrium and pisiform in the wrist (Fig. 1–2). The earliest erosive changes of any inflammatory arthropathy begin in these areas. Erosive changes occur between the triquetrium and pisiform before they occur around the ulnar styloid (Fig. 1–3). The Norgaard view will also reveal the reducible subluxations of inflammatory arthropathies and systemic lupus erythematosus, as the fingers are not rigidly positioned by the technician in this view (Fig. 1–4).

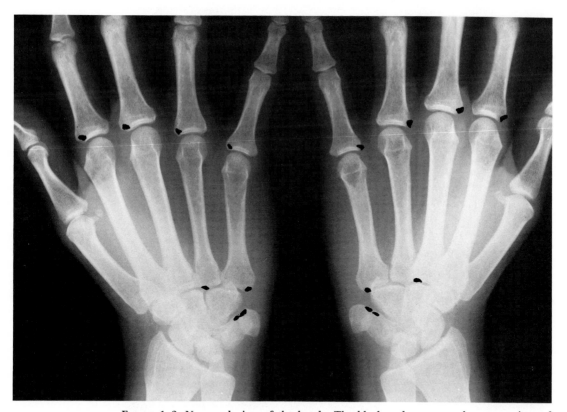

FIGURE 1–2. Norgaard view of the hands. The blackened areas are those areas imaged specifically on this view to demonstrate the earliest erosive changes in inflammatory disease. (From Brower AC: The radiologic approach to arthritis. Med Clin North Am 68:1593, 1984.)

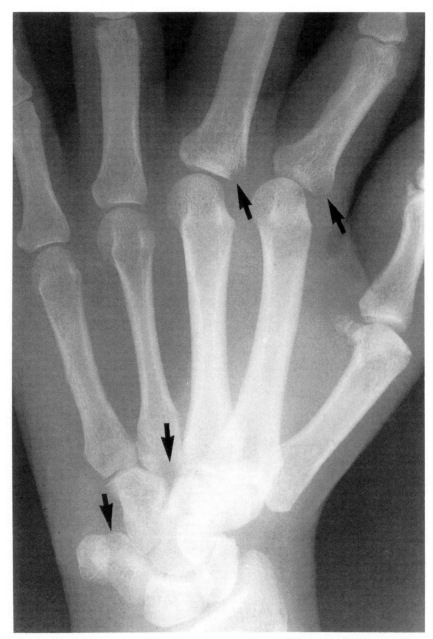

FIGURE 1–3. Norgaard view of the hand demonstrating early erosive changes at the base of the 2nd and 3rd proximal phalanges, the base of the 4th metacarpal, and the triquetrium as it articulates with the pisiform (arrows). (From Brower AC: The radiologic approach to arthritis. Med Clin North Am 68:1593, 1984.)

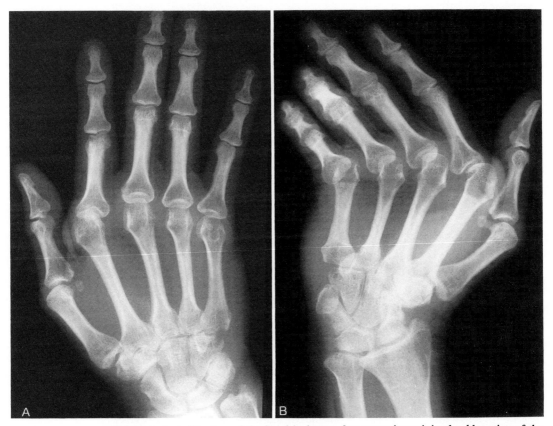

FIGURE 1–4. *A*, PA view of the hand in lupus, demonstrating minimal subluxation of the 2nd PIP and MCP joint. *B*, Norgaard view of the same hand in which the fingers are not rigidly positioned. Extensive subluxations become apparent.

2. Foot

The anteroposterior (AP) and lateral views of the foot are usually sufficient. One must be sure to obtain a high-quality radiograph of the calcaneus in the lateral view. Observation of the attachments of the plantar aponeurosis and Achilles tendon is important in many of the arthropathies (Fig. 1–5).

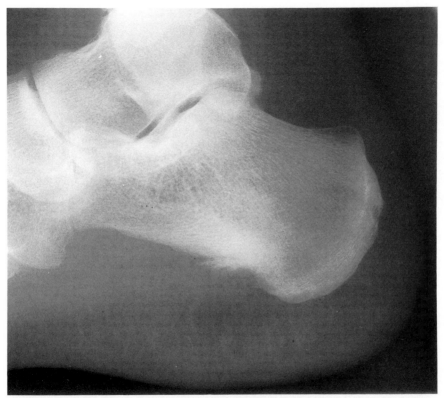

FIGURE 1–5. Lateral view of the calcaneus showing erosive change as well as bone productive change on the inferior aspect of the calcaneus at the attachment of the plantar aponeurosis. (From Brower AC: The radiographic features of psoriatic arthritis. *In* Gerber L, Espinoza L [eds]: Psoriatic Arthritis. Orlando, Grune & Stratton, 1985, p 125.)

3. Shoulder

Anteroposterior views of the shoulder should be obtained in true external and internal rotation. Erosive changes can usually be identified on at least one of these views. External rotation is best for demonstrating the presence of osteophytes. Internal rotation demonstrates the traumatic lesion of the Hill-Sachs deformity. Location of tendon calcification can be determined by observing change in the position of the calcification between internal and external rotation. The straight AP view does not image the true glenohumeral joint. In order for this joint to be imaged accurately, the patient should be placed in a 40-degree posterior oblique position (Fig. 1–6).

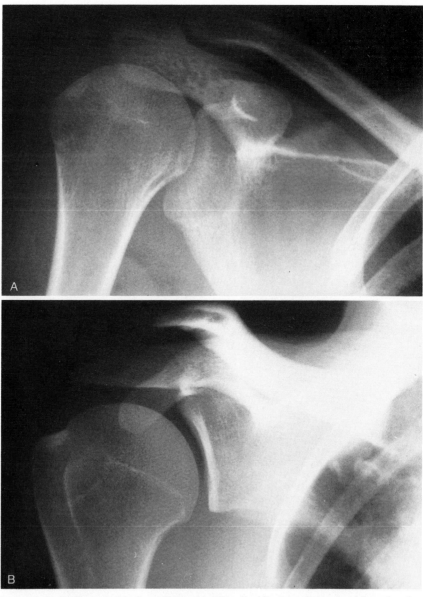

FIGURE 1–6. *A,* Normal AP view of the shoulder. *B,* AP view of the shoulder taken in a 40-degree posterior oblique position. This allows accurate evaluation of the glenohumeral joint.

4. Knee

The anteroposterior radiograph of the knee should be obtained in the standing position. This allows for accurate evaluation of loss of cartilage. If the patient is not standing, the medial and lateral compartments may appear perfectly normal (Fig. 1–7). In the standing position there may be asymmetry between the medial and lateral compartments, but unless the joint space measures less than 3 mm, cartilage loss is not the cause. The discrepancy between the compartments may be secondary to ligamentous instability. The standing AP view demonstrates displacement of the tibia on the femur and any pathological degree of varus or valgus angulation. The knee should also be radiographed in a nonstanding flexed lateral position. This allows evaluation of the patellofemoral joint space as well as identification of any abnormal position of the patella.

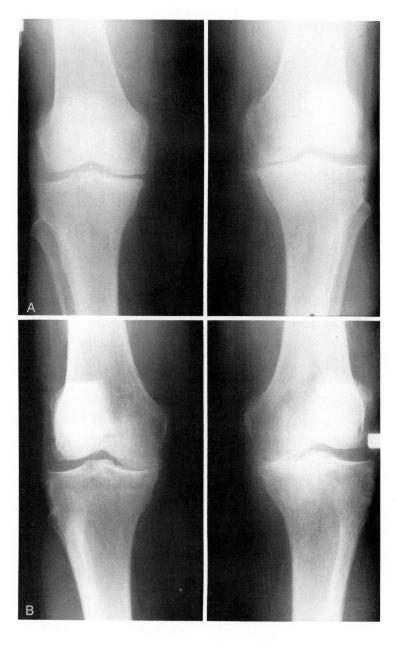

FIGURE 1–7. *A*, Table-top AP view of the knees. Despite the non–weight-bearing position, there is slight loss of the medial compartment of the left knee with secondary osteoarthritic changes. *B*, Standing AP view of the same knees. This view demonstrates total loss of the medial compartment of both knees.

5. Hip

The hip is usually radiographed in an AP and frogleg lateral position. In the AP view the hip is internally rotated to image the femoral neck to its fullest advantage. In the frogleg lateral view the hip is abducted. In this view the anterior and posterior portions of the femoral head are imaged. This view is most important in evaluating underlying osteonecrosis. While the entire head may appear to be involved on the AP view, the frogleg lateral view may demonstrate the abnormality to be limited to either the anterior or posterior section of the head. It is also the frogleg lateral view that demonstrates the subchondral lucency in osteonecrosis. In many patients, a vacuum phenomenon in the joint will be produced in the frogleg lateral view, helping to exclude the presence of synovial fluid. The vacuum phenomenon may also help in the evaluation of the cartilage present (Fig. 1–8).

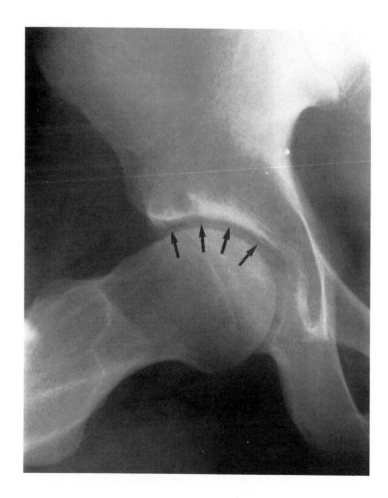

FIGURE 1–8. Frogleg lateral view of the hip. A vacuum phenomenon has been introduced into the joint space (arrows) and allows evaluation of the thickness of the cartilage present. The cartilage is thinner in the superolateral aspect of the hip joint.

6. Sacroiliac Joints

The modified Ferguson view is the only view necessary to evaluate the sacroiliac joints (Fig. 1–9). The patient is placed in a supine position and, when possible, the knees and hips are flexed. The x-ray tube is centered at L5-S1 and then angled 25 to 30 degrees toward the head. If it is angled too steeply, the pubic symphysis will overlie the sacroiliac joints and obscure them, preventing accurate evaluation. The modified Ferguson view brings into profile the anterior, inferior–most aspect of the sacroiliac joints. It is this part of the joint that is most frequently affected in any disorder of the sacroiliac joints. Ninety per cent of the time this view provides the clinician with an image that can be accurately evaluated. Conventional and computed tomography may be used if the pelvic soft tissues cause a problem on the plain film radiograph.

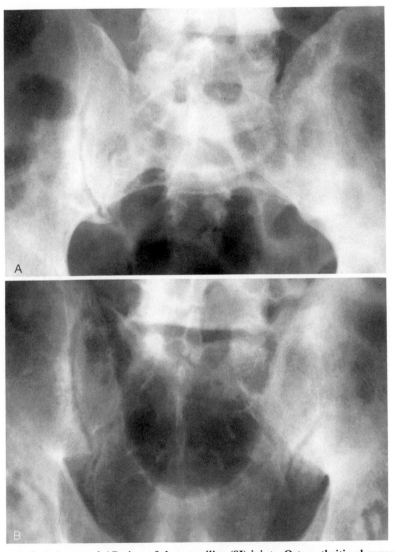

FIGURE 1–9. *A*, A normal AP view of the sacroiliac (SI) joints. Osteoarthritic changes are present in the right SI joint. The left SI joint appears ankylosed. *B*, AP Ferguson view of the same SI joints. The inferiormost aspect of the SI joint on the left side is normal; therefore, there is no ankylosis present. The apparent ankylosis is caused by a huge osteophyte that extends from the ilium across the SI joint to the sacrum. (From Brower AC: Disorders of the sacroiliac joint. Radiolog 1[20]:3, 1978.)

7. Cervical Spine

The lateral flexed view of the cervical spine is the single most important radiograph in the evaluation of cervical spine disease. Flexion opens the apophyseal joints and allows accurate observation of erosive disease. It demonstrates significant subluxation of one vertebral body on another. It also demonstrates abnormal laxity of the transverse ligament, which holds the odontoid adjacent to the atlas (Fig. 1–10). This finding is common in all inflammatory arthropathies but especially in rheumatoid arthritis.

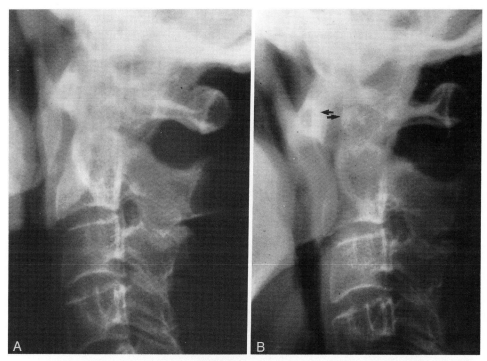

FIGURE 1–10. *A*, Lateral view of the upper cervical spine taken in a neutral position. There is no evidence of subluxation. *B*, Lateral view of the same cervical spine taken in flexion. The distance between the odontoid and the atlas has increased to greater than 3 mm (arrows). This indicates subluxation secondary to laxity of the transverse ligament.

The distribution of the joint involvement is key to the diagnosis of the specific arthropathy. Therefore, it is often necessary to obtain radiographs of more than just the symptomatic joint. Simple radiographic surveys can be performed, tailored to the working clinical diagnosis. For example, if ankylosing spondylitis is the working diagnosis, the survey should be tailored to the axial system; if rheumatoid arthritis is the working diagnosis, the survey should be tailored to the appendicular system. For the patient with vague articular complaints that fit no specific pattern, the following "poor man's" survey would be appropriate:

1. Posteroanterior and Norgaard views of both hands to include both wrists
2. Anteroposterior standing view of both knees
3. Anteroposterior view of the pelvis
4. Lateral flexed view of the cervical spine

This survey will provide sufficient diagnostic information, while exposing the patient to a relatively low dose of radiation at a reasonable cost.

CONVENTIONAL TOMOGRAPHY

Conventional tomography is used when the changes in the joint cannot be adequately visualized on the plain film. This lack of visualization is usually due to (1) the size of the joint, (2) the orientation of the joint, and, (3) most commonly, obscuration of the joint by the surrounding structures (Fig. 1–11). In the past, conventional tomography has been used almost routinely in imaging the sternoclavicular and temporomandibular joints. It has been used as an adjunct in imaging the sacroiliac joints and the occipito-atlanto-axial region of the cervical spine. Today computed tomography (CT) and/or magnetic resonance imaging (MRI) may be more useful. One must still consider cost and availability of these modalities. When conventional tomography is still used, zonography is suggested. This produces sections of increased thickness, but allows more contrast in the image.

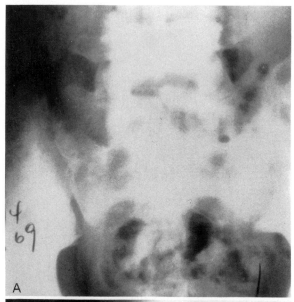

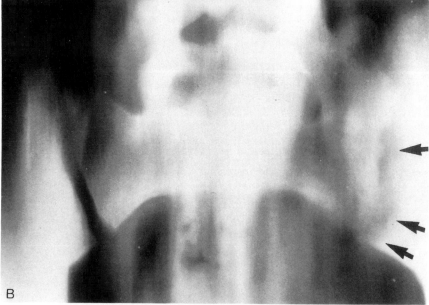

FIGURE 1–11. *A*, AP view of the sacroiliac joints. The right sacroiliac joint is normal. The left sacroiliac joint cannot be visualized because of the overlying soft tissue structures. *B*, Conventional tomography through the same sacroiliac joints. There is extensive erosive change involving the left sacroiliac joint (arrows). This proved to be a septic arthritis.

COMPUTED TOMOGRAPHY (CT)

Computed tomography does not play a primary role in the evaluation of articular disorders. The exquisite detail of erosive changes imaged on a technically well-done conventional radiograph is far superior to the bone detail observed on a computed tomography image. Physicians have recently advocated the use of computed tomography for the initial evaluation of sacroiliac disease. There are several reasons for this, including ease of positioning of the patient and ease of visualizing any abnormality imaged. There is an art to obtaining a high-quality conventional radiograph and an art to its interpretation. When appropriately performed, conventional radiography is still the modality of choice. It images earlier changes and costs far less. Considering its high cost, its inability to image subtle change, and the limited availability of machine time, computed tomography should be used only as an adjunct to plain film radiography.

Two areas in which computed tomography excels in the evaluation of articular diseases are the evaluation of osteonecrosis of the femoral head and the diagnosis of pseudotumors of hemophilia. In the work-up of osteonecrosis of the femoral head, computed tomography helps the surgeon in understanding the geography of the necrotic area (Fig. 1–12). In the evaluation of the pseudotumor of hemophilia, again computed tomography demonstrates the geography of the tumor—its contour and its relationship to adjacent structures. Imaging of its internal consistency may help resolve a diagnostic dilemma.

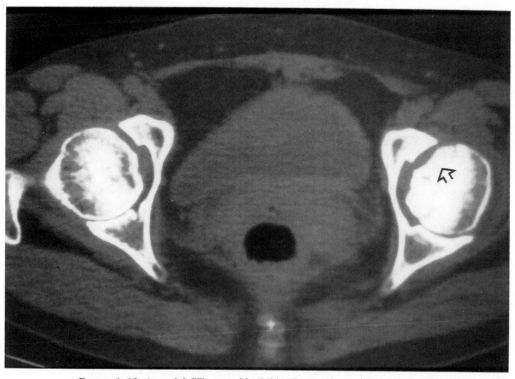

FIGURE 1–12. An axial CT scan of both hips in a patient with osteonecrosis. Although the diagnosis of osteonecrosis could be made from the conventional radiograph, this image demonstrates that the location of the subchondral fragment is anterior (arrow). (Courtesy of Dr. P. L. Choyke, Georgetown University Hospital, Washington, D.C.)

BONE SCINTIGRAPHY

Bone scintigraphy may be extremely helpful in the evaluation of the patient with articular disease. It is useful in three ways: (1) it may confirm the presence of disease; (2) it may demonstrate the distribution of disease; (3) it may help to evaluate the activity of the disease. Bone scintigraphy is by far the most sensitive indicator of active disease. It will confirm the presence of hyperemia in inflammation that may not be apparent radiographically. With careful observation of a high-resolution image of a joint, one may determine the exact location of the active disease. One may be able to distinguish a tendinitis from a synovitis, or a synovitis from a primary bone lesion.

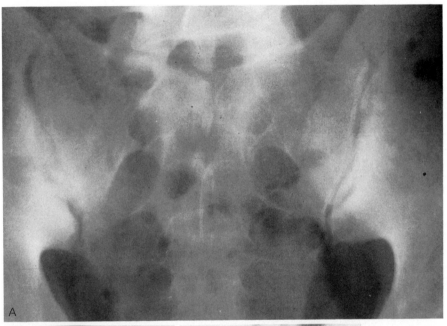

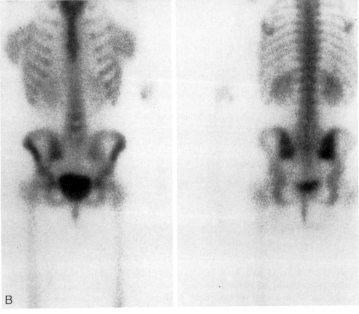

FIGURE 1–13. *A*, AP Ferguson view of the sacroiliac joints demonstrating erosive disease with repair involving the right sacroiliac joint. The left sacroiliac joint appears normal. Unilateral involvement of the right sacroiliac joint is most consistent with infection. *B*, Bone scan of the same patient demonstrating increased activity in both sacroiliac joints. This would indicate involvement of the radiographically normal left SI joint and change the diagnosis from infection to early Reiter's disease.

While confirming abnormality in one joint, observation of increased activity in other areas of the body may help in making the correct diagnosis. An excellent example is the young adult who shows radiographic erosive changes in one sacroiliac joint. If bone scintigraphy shows increased uptake in that one sacroiliac joint only, infection becomes the working diagnosis. However, if bone scintigraphy shows increased uptake in both sacroiliac joints, Reiter's disease becomes the working diagnosis (Fig. 1–13). The distribution of the uptake within the hand may distinguish rheumatoid arthritis from erosive osteoarthritis in the elderly female (Fig. 1–14).

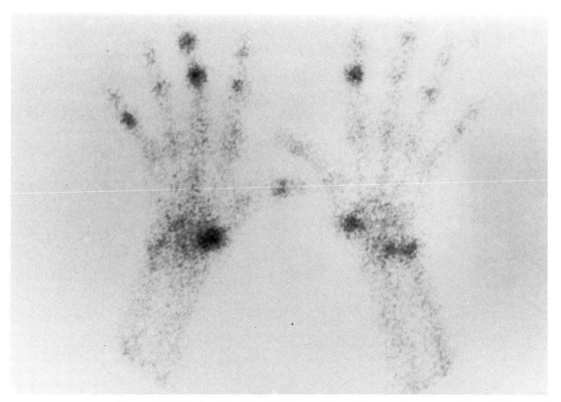

FIGURE 1–14. Technetium-99m MDP scan of hands in a post-menopausal female. Increased uptake of the tracer is observed on the left in the 2nd, 3rd, and 5th PIP joints, the 3rd DIP joint, the 1st carpometacarpal joint, and the greater multangular-navicular joint; on the right in the 2nd PIP joint and the 1st carpometacarpal joint. This distribution is consistent with erosive osteoarthritis. (Courtesy of Dr. J. Balseiro, Georgetown University Hospital, Washington, D. C.)

Serial bone scintigraphy has also been helpful in evaluating the activity of disease at a particular point in time. It may differentiate active disease from disease in remission. In osteonecrosis specifically, it may demonstrate the infarctive stage, the reparative stage, and the inactive stage (Fig. 1–15). Bone scintigraphy should be considered an integral part of the evaluation of the patient with articular disease.

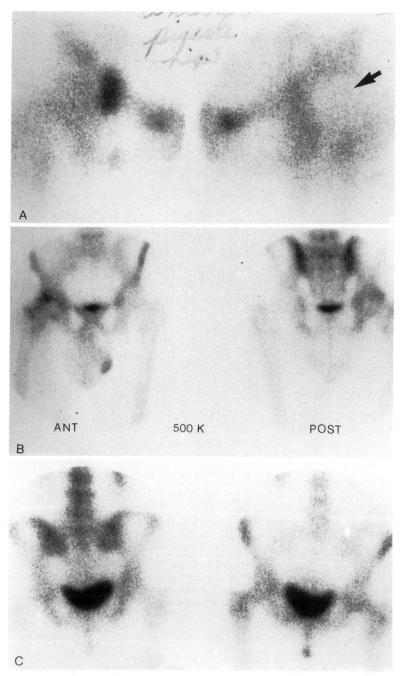

FIGURE 1–15. **Technetium-99m MDP scans of hips in different stages of osteonecrosis.** *A,* **Infarctive stage—hip 24 hours after a subcapital fracture demonstrating no tracer uptake in the left femoral head (arrow). Increased uptake is present in pubic rami fractures.** *B,* **Reparative stage—increased tracer uptake in the right hip, with a central area of decreased uptake.** *C,* **Inactive stage—normal tracer uptake in both hips, which radiographically demonstrate advanced changes of osteonecrosis.**

ULTRASONOGRAPHY

Ultrasonography is of limited use in the evaluation of articular disease. It was first used to evaluate the presence of a Baker's cyst in the patient who had either a palpable popliteal mass or symptoms of thrombophlebitis due to extravasation of cyst material into the adjacent muscle (Fig. 1–16). It is the preferred modality for imaging this problem because of its non-invasive nature. Ultrasonography has also been useful in evaluating pseudotumors of hemophilia, aiding in diagnosis and providing visualization of the geography of the tumor. Since ultrasound is less invasive than computed tomography, it is the modality of choice. Recently physicians have been using ultrasound successfully in evaluating rotator cuff tears. However, this modality should be used only when the ultrasonographer has a clear understanding of the anatomy in this area and experience in interpreting the findings. Arthrography may have to be performed if ultrasonography does not provide a clear diagnosis.

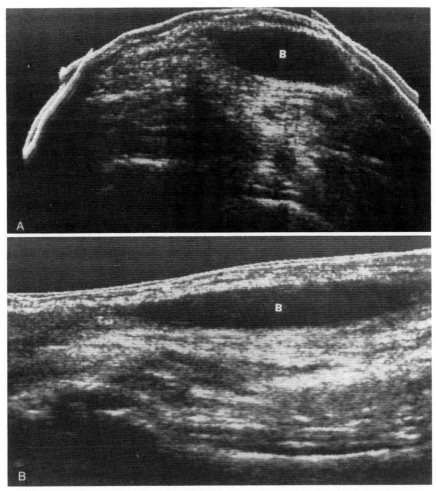

FIGURE 1–16. Transverse (A) and longitudinal (B) static scans through the upper left calf. A large superficial, anechoic mass is present. The well-defined fusiform appearance is typical of Baker's cyst (B). (From Grant EG, Earll J, Richardson JE, Dunne A: High-resolution real-time sonography: The study of superficial body parts. Med Clin North Am 68:1609, 1984.)

MAGNETIC RESONANCE IMAGING (MRI)

The role of magnetic resonance imaging has yet to be defined for use in articular disease. It is far too young a modality to know at this point how and where it will be useful. At the present time, magnetic resonance does not image bone; therefore, if demonstration and documentation of changes in bone are important to the clinician, this modality should not be chosen. Magnetic resonance images medullary contents of bone, articular cartilage, fibrocartilage, muscles, tendons, and fat. Each of these can be separated from the others owing to differences in signal intensity, thus allowing excellent image contrast.

Today the articular-related disease that has received the most attention is osteonecrosis. Magnetic resonance appears to be the most sensitive modality in detecting osteonecrosis (Fig. 1–17). There have been reports that MRI has detected osteonecrosis before bone scintigraphy. Unfortunately, while MRI has proved to be very sensitive, it has also proved to be non-specific. The tendency has been to overdiagnose, identifying any change in signal intensity in the femoral head as osteonecrosis. The clinician must be aware of this tendency when employing MRI and carefully correlate the abnormality with the clinical picture.

Some work has been done on imaging cartilage disorders. Hyaline cartilage can be distinguished from fibrocartilage; hyaline cartilage gives an intermediate signal, whereas fibrocartilage gives a lower intensity signal. Irregularity and thinning of cartilage have been demonstrated on MRI. Hyaline cartilage of non-ossified epiphyses has been imaged in children; this may help in the future in evaluation of juvenile chronic arthritis. In the future MRI may provide identification of the substances deposited into cartilage.

Since magnetic resonance images ligaments and tendons, work now is being done on evaluating chronic rotator cuff tears. Improvements need to be made before this becomes the modality of choice.

Synovium and synovial effusions have been imaged by magnetic resonance. Hypertrophy and irregularity of the synovium have been demonstrated, which may become important in the evaluation of inflammatory arthropathies. Effusions are imaged as low signal intensity on T_1 weighted images and high signal intensity on T_2 weighted images. However, at this time, it has been impossible to determine the nature of the effusion. It does appear possible to distinguish the synovium from the effusion itself.

The greatest work in magnetic resonance imaging has been done in the spine. Papers are forthcoming on the evaluation of spinal cord abnormalities in the cervical area in patients with rheumatoid arthritis. MRI is most likely to become the modality of choice in evaluating rheumatoid patients with neurological symptoms. MRI is also becoming the modality of choice in evaluation of temporomandibular joint arthritis.

While still young, magnetic resonance imaging promises in the future to play an important role in the evaluation of the patient with articular disease. However, there must first be improved image resolution, improved image acquisition time, decreased image cost, and increased experience in image interpretation.

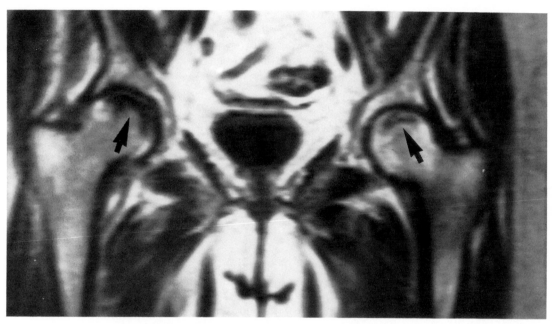

FIGURE 1–17. Coronal MR scan in a patient with SLE. Crescent-shaped areas of decreased signal intensity represent changes of osteonecrosis (arrows). (Courtesy of Dr. B. Pastakia, National Institutes of Health, Bethesda, MD.)

SUGGESTED READINGS

Bretzke CA, Crass JR, Craig EV, Feinberg SB: Ultrasonography of the rotator cuff: Normal and pathologic anatomy. Invest Radiol 20:311–315, 1985.

Brower AC: Disorders of the sacroiliac joint. Radiolog 1 (20):3–25, 1978.

Gillespy T III, Genant H, Helms CA: Magnetic resonance imaging of osteonecrosis. Radiol Clin North Am 24:193–208, 1986.

Goldberg RP, Genant HK, Shimshak R, Shames D: Applications and limitations of quantitative sacroiliac joint scintigraphy. Radiology 128:683, 1978.

Helms CA, Gillespy T III, Sims RE, Richardson ML: Magnetic resonance imaging of internal derangement of the temporomandibular joint. Radiol Clin North Am 24:189–192, 1986.

Kumari S, Fulco JD, Karayalcin G, Lipton R: Gray scale ultrasound: Evaluation of iliopsoas hematomas in hemophiliacs. AJR 133:103, 1979.

Leach RE, Gregg T, Ferris JS: Weight-bearing radiography in osteoarthritis of the knee. Radiology 97:265, 1970.

Martel W, Poznanski AK: The effect of traction on the hip in osteonecrosis. A comment on the "radiolucent crescent line." Radiology 94:505, 1970.

Moore CP, Sarti DA, Louie JS: Ultrasonographic demonstration of popliteal cysts in rheumatoid arthritis: A non-invasive technique. Arthritis Rheum 18:577, 1975.

Norgaard F: Earliest roentgenological changes in polyarthritis of the rheumatoid type: Rheumatoid arthritis. Radiology 85:325, 1965.

Sims RE, Genant HK: Magnetic resonance imaging of joint disease. Radiol Clin North Am 24:179–188, 1986.

Slivka J, Resnick D: An improved radiographic view of the glenohumeral joint. J Can Assoc Radiol 30:83, 1979.

Sy WM, Bay R, Camera A: Hand images: Normal and abnormal. J Nucl Med 18:419, 1977.

Weissberg DL, Resnick D, Taylor A, et al.: Rheumatoid arthritis and its variants: Analysis of scintiphotographic, radiographic, and clinical examinations. AJR 131:665, 1978.

Part I

APPROACH TO RADIOGRAPHIC CHANGES OBSERVED IN A SPECIFIC JOINT

chapter 2

EVALUATION OF THE HAND FILM

Radiographs of the hands are probably the most informative part of any screening series for arthritis. It is suggested that two views be obtained for evaluation: a PA view and a Norgaard view of both hands and wrists (see Chapter 1). The former is excellent for imaging mineralization and soft tissue swelling; the latter is necessary for imaging early erosive changes. Using these two views, a systematic approach to observation should be employed. One must observe (1) the radiographic changes occurring in a specific joint and (2) the distribution of these changes within the hand and wrist in order to make an accurate diagnosis.

RADIOGRAPHIC CHANGES

The radiographic changes occurring around a specific joint to be evaluated are soft tissue swelling, subluxation/dislocation, mineralization, calcification, joint space narrowing, erosion, and bone production. Each arthropathy has its own characteristic set of changes.

23

Soft Tissue Swelling

1. SYMMETRICAL SWELLING AROUND AN INVOLVED JOINT (FIG. 2–1)

This is most easily evaluated around the IP joints and wrist. Evaluation of the MCP joints often requires low kilovoltage soft tissue technique. This type of swelling may be seen in any of the inflammatory arthropathies but is most common in rheumatoid arthritis.

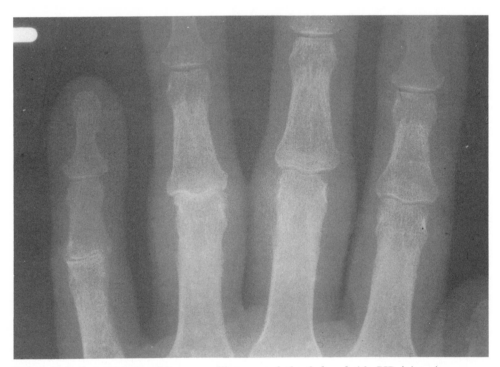

FIGURE 2–1. Symmetrical soft-tissue swelling around the 3rd and 4th PIP joints in rheumatoid arthritis.

2. ASYMMETRICAL SWELLING AROUND AN INVOLVED JOINT (FIG. 2–2)

This may not be actual soft tissue swelling, but rather soft tissue asymmetry due to subluxation and/or an osteophyte. The osteophyte may have a non-opaque cartilage cap that distorts the soft tissue. This swelling is seen in osteoarthritis and erosive osteoarthritis.

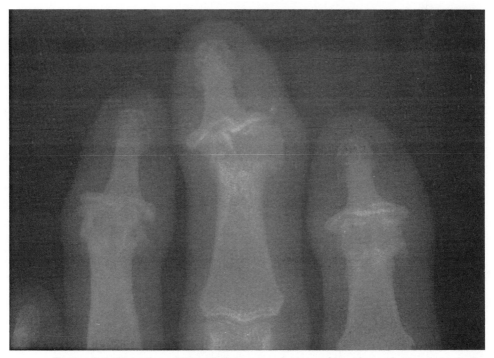

FIGURE 2–2. Distortion of the soft tissue secondary to subluxation and osteophytes in the DIP joints of a patient with osteoarthritis.

3. DIFFUSE FUSIFORM SWELLING OF AN ENTIRE DIGIT (FIG. 2–3)

This swollen digit is reminiscent of a sausage or a cocktail hot dog. This type of swelling is seen commonly in psoriatic arthritis and in Reiter's syndrome when it involves the hand.

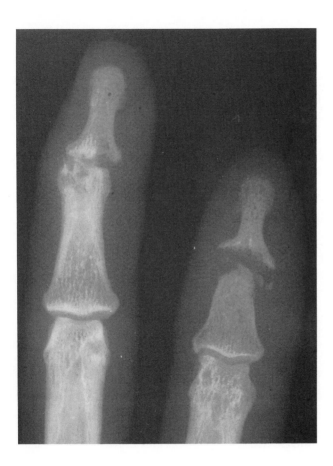

FIGURE 2–3. Swollen digit resembling a sausage in psoriatic arthritis.

4. LUMPY, BUMPY SOFT TISSUE SWELLING (FIG. 2–4)

This is produced by infiltration with a substance foreign to the normal tissues around the joint, i.e., urate crystals, xanthomatous tissue, or amyloid. An eccentric bump may be observed near or away from the joint. Such a swelling is most commonly seen in gout and rarely in xanthomatous or amyloid disease.

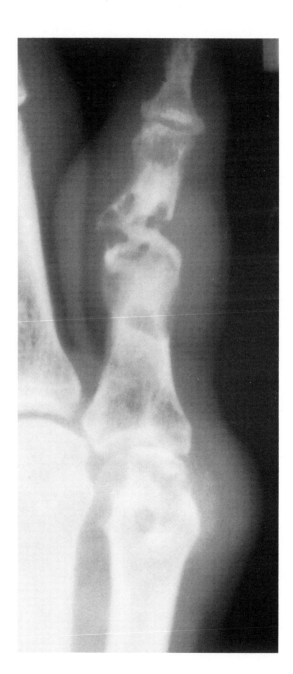

FIGURE 2–4. Soft tissue masses distributed asymmetrically around the PIP and MCP joints of the 5th digit in gout.

Subluxation

Subluxations may not be visualized on the PA view of the hands and wrists, for the technician will reduce any subluxation during positioning. Subluxations become apparent on the Norgaard view, for the fingers are not supported in a fixed position. Subluxation is a prominent feature of rheumatoid arthritis and the arthritis of lupus. The proximal phalanges sublux in an ulnar and palmar direction in relationship to the adjacent metacarpals (Fig. 2–5). One can distinguish the arthritis of lupus from rheumatoid arthritis in that erosive disease is not present in the former. Subluxations do occur in osteoarthritis. These are usually in a lateral direction, deviating either radially or ulnarly (Fig. 2–6).

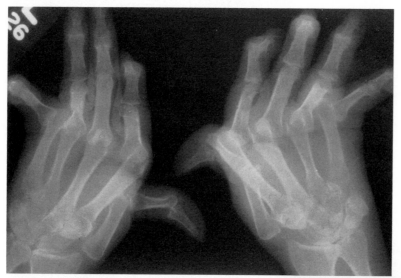

FIGURE 2–5. Subluxations of the proximal phalanges in an ulnar and palmar direction in relationship to the adjacent metacarpals in lupus arthritis. Ulnar subluxation of carpals. Hyperextension of PIP's and flexion deformities of DIP's.

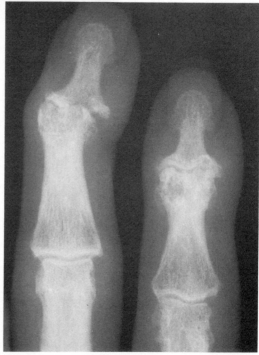

FIGURE 2–6. Lateral subluxation of the distal phalanx in relationship to the middle phalanx of the 3rd digit in osteoarthritis.

Mineralization

Overall mineralization is evaluated by observing the metacarpal shaft of the 2nd or the 3rd digit. The sum of the two cortices of the shaft should equal one half the width of the shaft in a normally mineralized digit (Fig. 2–7). The degree of generalized osteoporosis can be accurately judged by the sum of the two cortices in relationship to the width of the shaft (Fig. 2–8).

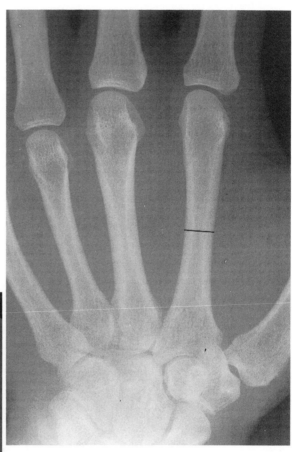

FIGURE 2–7. Shaft of the 2nd metacarpal demonstrating normal mineralization. At the line drawn on the diaphysis, the sum of the two cortices equals half the width of the shaft. (From Brower AC: The radiologic approach to arthritis. Med Clin North Am 68:1593, 1984.)

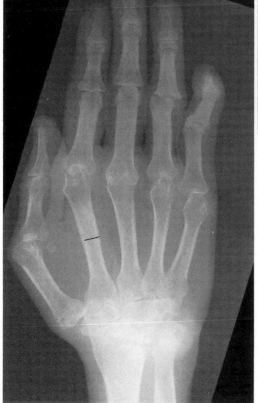

FIGURE 2–8. Diffuse osteoporosis. At the line drawn on the diaphysis of the 2nd metacarpal, the sum of the two cortices is clearly less than half the width of the shaft. (From Kantor S, Brower AC: Radiographic assessment. *In* Rothermich N, Whisler R: Rheumatoid Arthritis. Orlando, FL, Grune & Stratton, Inc, 1985, p 57.)

1. NORMAL MINERALIZATION (FIG. 2–7)

This is typical of every arthropathy except rheumatoid arthritis. The maintenance of normal mineralization helps to distinguish the "rheumatoid variants"—psoriasis, Reiter's syndrome, and ankylosing spondylitis—from rheumatoid arthritis. The crystalline arthropathies and the osteoarthropathies maintain normal mineralization.

2. JUXTA-ARTICULAR DEMINERALIZATION

This change has no objective criteria. The metaphyseal-epiphyseal part of the digit is always less dense than the diaphysis, for the cortical bone is thinner in the metaphysis and epiphysis. Dramatic differences are easy to see (Fig. 2–9). However, juxta-articular osteoporosis is a nonspecific finding; it is observed in many abnormal conditions, including post-traumatic change. It may be present in any of the arthropathies at any time. Observation of its presence only helps to establish that something is abnormal in the hand.

3. DIFFUSE OSTEOPOROSIS (FIG. 2–8)

This change is associated only with rheumatoid arthritis. It is seen in the advanced stages of this disease. All other arthropathies tend to maintain normal mineralization. If one observes osteoporosis in a patient with another arthropathy, such as gout, the generalized osteoporosis may be secondary to medication or to the normal aging process. It should not be blamed primarily on the arthropathy.

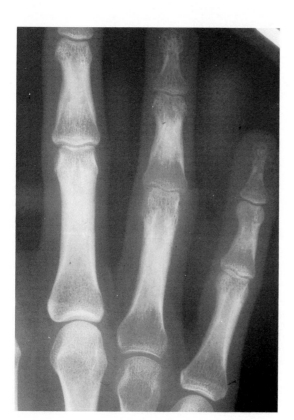

FIGURE 2–9. Juxta-articular osteoporosis of the MCP and IP joints of the 4th and 5th digits in rheumatoid arthritis.

Calcification

1. SOFT TISSUE MASS CALCIFICATION (FIG. 2–10)

The urate crystals of gout are not radiopaque. However, when the urate crystals deposit in the soft tissues to form a tophus, calcium is precipitated with the urate crystals to varying degrees. Therefore the tophus may be just slightly denser than the surrounding soft tissue structures or it may be very densely calcified. In either case, such a tophus is part of the radiographic picture of gout.

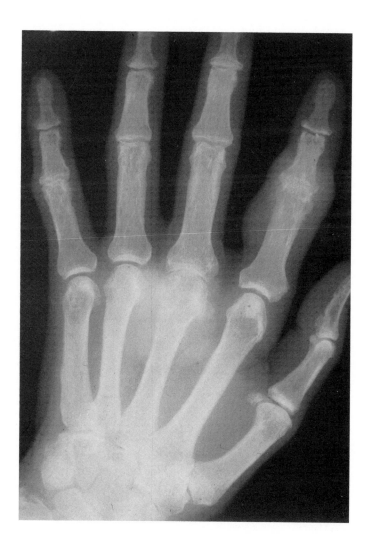

FIGURE 2–10. Calcification in a soft tissue mass or tophus surrounding the 3rd MCP joint. Less dense tophi in the 2nd digit in gout.

2. CARTILAGE CALCIFICATION (CHONDROCALCINOSIS) (FIG. 2–11)

Calcium pyrophosphate crystals deposit in hyaline and fibrous cartilage, producing a radiographic picture of calcified cartilage. When seen in two or more joints (meaning one knee and one wrist, not two knees), the radiographic diagnosis of calcium pyrophosphate deposition disease (CPPD) can be made. In the older literature, "chondrocalcinosis" was associated with a long list of diseases. For example, it was listed as a manifestation of gout. However, it is now known that while urate crystals deposited in soft tissues may precipitate calcium, urate crystals deposited in cartilage will not precipitate calcium. Therefore, a patient with known gout who demonstrates calcification of hyaline or fibrous cartilage must also have deposition of calcium pyrophosphate crystals in the cartilage; thus the patient has both gout and CPPD. The only two diseases known to cause actual deposition of calcium pyrophosphate crystals in cartilage, other than idiopathic CPPD, are hyperparathyroidism and hemochromatosis.

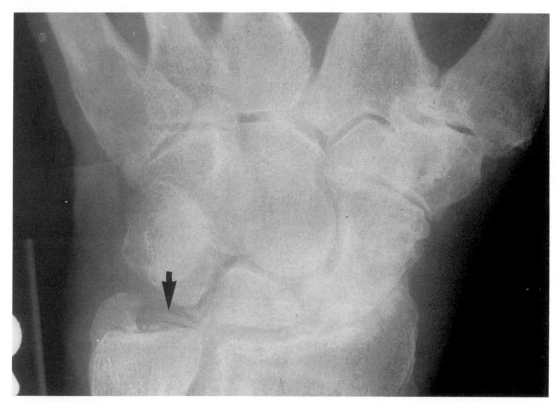

FIGURE 2–11. Calcification in the triangular fibrocartilage of the wrist (arrow).

3. TENDINOUS AND SOFT TISSUE CALCIFICATION (FIG. 2–12)

Hydroxyapatite crystals deposit in tendons and bursae, producing the classic tendinitis or bursitis of the shoulder. The second most common location for this deposition is over the greater trochanter. It can also cause a problem around the elbow or the wrist. Hydroxyapatite is also known to deposit in soft tissues in various systemic diseases, such as scleroderma, dermatomyositis, renal osteodystrophy, etc. However, patients have presented recently with hydroxyapatite deposition in numerous tendinous and soft tissue sites without an underlying systemic disease. Associated with this deposition, erosive changes of the small joints of the hand have developed (Fig. 2–13). This disease entity has become known as hydroxyapatite deposition disease, or HADD.

FIGURE 2–12. Hydroxyapatite deposition into a tendon.
→

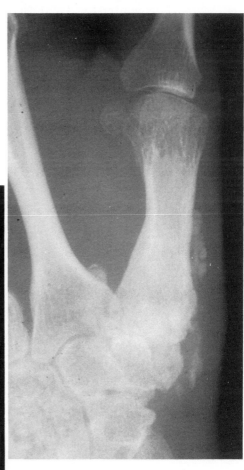

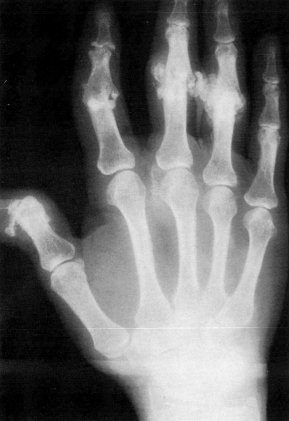

←
FIGURE 2–13. Hydroxyapatite deposition into soft tissues surrounding PIP joints with erosive changes of the joints in a patient with hydroxyapatite deposition disease. (Courtesy of Dr. M. K. Dalinka, Hospital of the University of Pennsylvania, Philadelphia.)

Joint Space Narrowing

1. MAINTENANCE OF JOINT SPACE

While urate crystals may deposit within the cartilage of a joint and cause secondary loss of the joint space, gout is one of the few arthropathies that can cause significant changes around the joint while maintaining the joint space itself. A tophus deposited on the extensor aspect of a joint may cause significant erosive change of the dorsal aspect of the joint while preserving the flexor aspect (Fig. 2–14). Radiographically one may observe extensive erosion with a ghost of a joint space imaging through the erosion. In the rare instance of pigmented villonodular synovitis involving the wrist, the involved joint will usually be maintained.

2. UNIFORM NARROWING (FIG. 2–15)

All of the arthropathies except for osteoarthritis produce uniform narrowing of the joint space. This includes the inflammatory arthropathies that erode the cartilage and all other arthropathies that deposit extra substance into the cartilage, i.e., the crystalline arthropathies, acromegaly, and Wilson's disease.

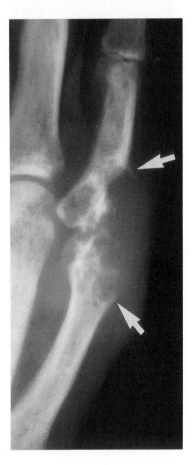

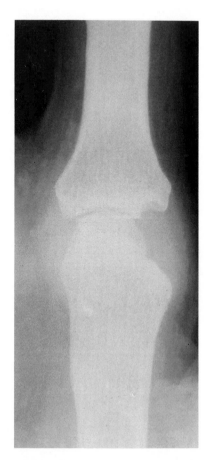

FIGURE 2–14. Extensive erosion of the dorsal aspect of the MCP joint, sparing the volar aspect of the joint. Erosive changes extend a considerable distance from the joint. Note sclerotic borders to erosions and the overhanging edge of cortex (arrows). The changes are typical of gout.

FIGURE 2–15. Uniform narrowing of an MCP joint in rheumatoid arthritis. Note also STS and erosion. (Courtesy of R. G. Dussault, Hotel-Dieu de Montreal, Canada.)

3. NON-UNIFORM NARROWING (FIG. 2–16)

This is typical of osteoarthritis and erosive osteoarthritis.

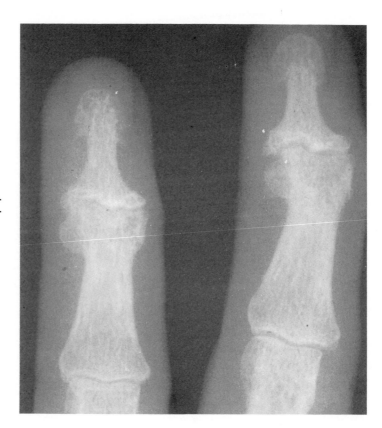

FIGURE 2–16. Non-uniform narrowing of the DIP joints in osteoarthritis.

Erosion

1. AGGRESSIVE EROSIONS

These are erosions that are actively changing while the radiograph is being taken. They have no sclerotic borders or evidence of reparative bone. In the inflammatory arthritides, early erosions are seen in the "bare" areas of bone. The "bare" area is located within the joint, between the edge of the articular cartilage and the attachment of the synovium. The very first radiographic change is a disruption of the white cortical line in the bare area, giving a "dot-dash" appearance (Fig. 2–17). These early erosions are best seen in the metacarpal heads or on the Norgaard view at the base of the proximal phalanges on the radial side (Fig. 2–18). As these erosions progress, they involve more and more of the joint, ignoring the original barrier of cartilage (Fig. 2–19). Eventually the entire joint may be destroyed. The end of the proximal bone may be eroded in such a fashion as to appear whittled or pointed while the end of the adjacent distal bone becomes splayed or cup-like (Fig. 2–20). This type of erosion has been called a pencil-in-cup deformity and is most commonly seen with psoriatic arthritis.

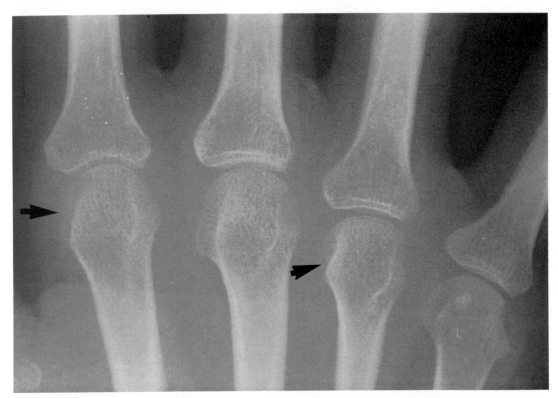

FIGURE 2–17. Disruption of the white cortical line on the radial aspect of the heads of the 2nd and 4th metacarpals (arrows). These are early aggressive erosions in the bare areas of the metacarpal head in rheumatoid arthritis.

FIGURE 2–18. Erosion of the base of the proximal phalanx on the radial aspect in a patient with rheumatoid arthritis (arrow). There is also adjacent erosion of the metacarpal head.

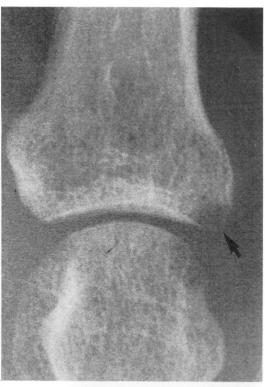

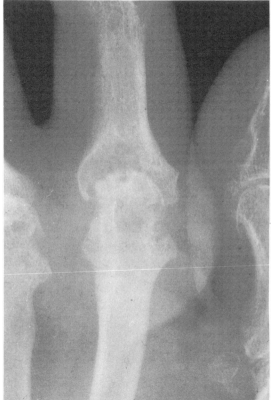

FIGURE 2–19. Extensive erosion of the MCP joint in a patient with rheumatoid arthritis.

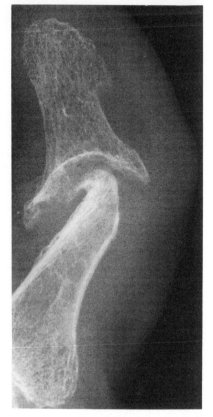

FIGURE 2–20. "Pencil-in-cup" erosive change of the IP joint of the thumb in psoriatic arthritis.

2. NON-AGGRESSIVE EROSIONS

These erosions have a fine sclerotic border outlining the edge of the erosion. In the case of the inflammatory arthritides, this is a sign that repair has occurred or that the disease is in remission (Fig. 2–21). In other arthropathies it indicates the indolence of the erosion (Fig. 2–22). It is most commonly seen in gout. Such an erosion is caused by an adjacent tophus. The bone changes caused by the tophus occur extremely slowly and at such a rate that the bone has time to respond and repair.

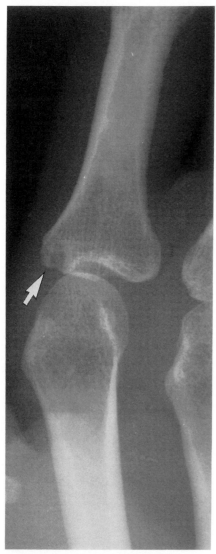
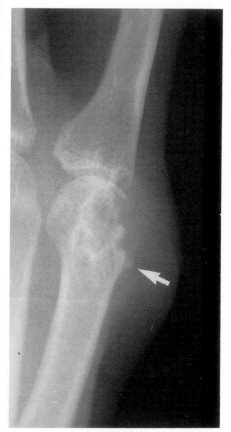

FIGURE 2–21   FIGURE 2–22

FIGURE 2–21. Sclerotic border to an erosion at the base of the proximal phalanx of the 2nd MCP joint in rheumatoid arthritis in remission (arrow).

FIGURE 2–22. Large erosions with sclerotic borders involving the MCP joint of the 5th digit in gout. Overhanging edge of the cortex is evident (arrow). (From Brower AC: The radiologic approach to arthritis. Med Clin North Am 68:1593, 1984.)

3. LOCATION

The location of the erosion within a specific joint is important in distinguishing one arthropathy from another. The erosions of an inflammatory arthropathy occur at the margins of the joint. The erosions of erosive osteoarthritis tend to occur in the central portion of the joint. In diagnosing distal interphalangeal (DIP) joint disease, the erosive pattern is all-important. The marginal erosions of psoriasis have been compared to "mouse-ears" (Fig. 2–23), and the central erosion of erosive osteoarthritis has been compared to a "seagull" (Fig. 2–24). The erosions of gout may occur away from the joint or on one side of the joint, leaving the rest of the joint intact (Fig. 2–14).

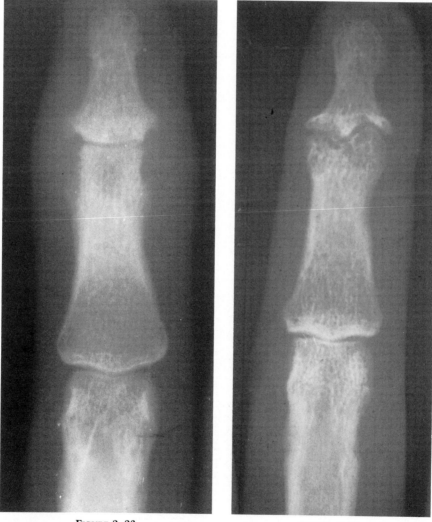

FIGURE 2–23   FIGURE 2–24

FIGURE 2–23. Marginal erosions resembling "mouse-ears" in the DIP joint of a patient with psoriatic arthritis. (From Brower AC: The radiographic features of psoriatic arthritis. *In* Gerber L, Espinoza L (eds): Psoriatic Arthritis. Orlando, FL, Grune & Stratton, Inc, 1985, p 125.)

FIGURE 2–24. Central erosion combined with osteophytes to create a "seagull" appearance in the DIP joint of a patient with erosive osteoarthritis.

Bone Production

1. PERIOSTEAL NEW BONE FORMATION

This is new bone that is deposited along the shaft of the phalanx or in the metaphysis just behind an erosion (Fig. 2–25). Initially this response is exuberant and fluffy in appearance but with time becomes incorporated into the parent bone as solid bone formation (Fig. 2–26). This may lead to the appearance of a widened phalanx. This type of new bone formation is characteristic of psoriatic arthritis, and Reiter's arthritis when it involves a hand. It is a feature that distinguishes the spondyloarthropathies from rheumatoid arthritis.

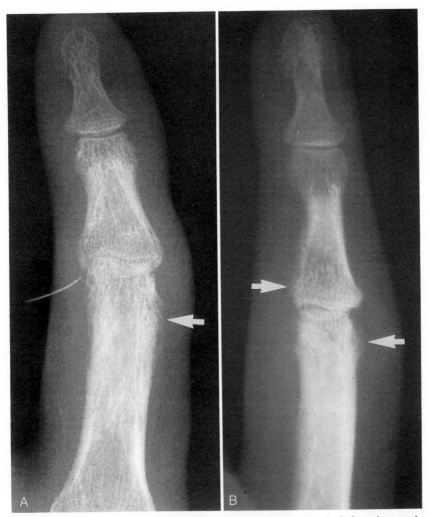

FIGURE 2–25. *A,* Periosteal reaction along the shaft of the proximal phalanx in a patient with psoriatic arthritis. *B,* New bone formation behind erosive changes involving the PIP joint in a patient with psoriatic arthritis (arrows).

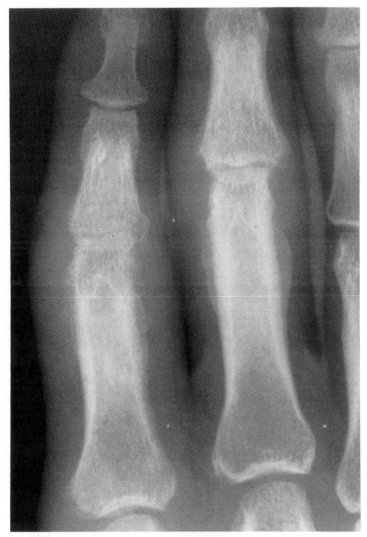

FIGURE 2–26. Solid periosteal new bone formation along the shafts of the 2nd and 3rd proximal phalanges in a patient with psoriatic arthritis.

2. Bone Ankylosis

This is bony bridging of a joint and is seen only in arthropathies that aggressively destroy the cartilage of the joint. It is therefore seen primarily in the inflammatory arthropathies. In rheumatoid arthritis bone ankylosis will occur in the carpal area but will not occur distal to the carpal area. In the spondyloarthropathies, bone ankylosis will occur not only in the carpals but in the IP joints. This is another distinguishing feature in separating the spondyloarthropathies from rheumatoid arthritis. Bone ankylosis will occur in erosive osteoarthritis, because of its inflammatory component, but not in primary osteoarthritis (Fig. 2–27). Bone ankylosis is not a feature of the crystalline arthropathies.

3. Overhanging Edge of Cortex

This is a characteristic of a chronic indolent type of erosion and therefore is seen most commonly in gout. As the tophus erodes into the bone the edge of the cortex is lifted or pushed outward, producing an overhanging edge (Figs. 2–14 and 2–22). This characteristic is seen in at least 40 per cent of the erosions produced in gout.

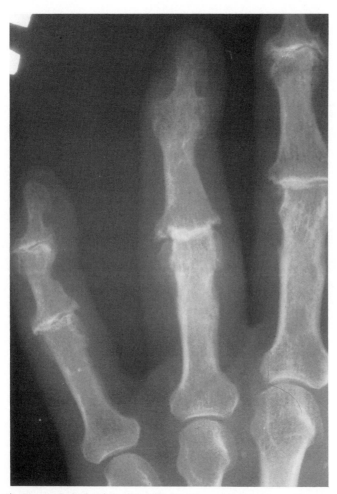

FIGURE 2–27. Bone ankylosis of the 4th DIP joint in a patient with erosive osteoarthritis.

4. SUBCHONDRAL BONE (FIG. 2–28)

This is reparative bone laid down just beneath the white cortical line. It occurs with degeneration or slow loss of cartilage and is a hallmark of osteoarthritis. However, it is also a feature of the crystalline arthropathies or any arthropathy in which a substance is deposited in the cartilage and secondary loss occurs. This type of bone production is not seen in the inflammatory arthropathies unless the disease is in a state of remission.

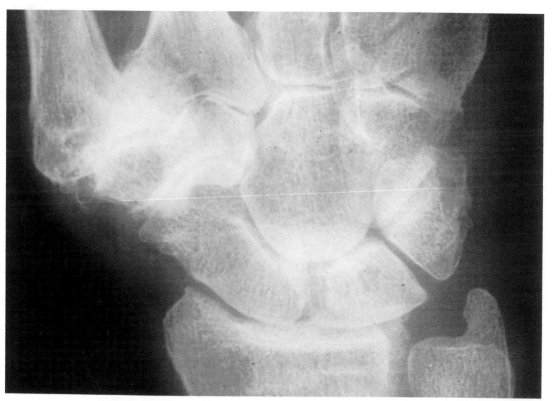

FIGURE 2–28. Subchondral sclerosis and joint space narrowing between the base of the 1st metacarpal, greater multangular, and distal navicular bones in a patient with osteoarthritis.

5. Osteophytes (Figs. 2–2, 2–6, and 2–16)

Osteophytes are bone extensions of a normal articular surface. They occur where the adjacent cartilage has undergone degeneration and subsequent loss. On the lateral radiograph, the osteophytes at the articular surfaces of the phalanges extend toward the body (Fig. 2–29). Osteophytes formed on metacarpal heads extend in a palmar direction and, on the PA view, resemble hooks (Fig. 2–30). Osteophytes are a hallmark of osteoarthritis. However, they are also a feature of any arthropathy that leads to slow degeneration or loss of cartilage, i.e., the crystalline arthropathies and acromegaly.

FIGURE 2–29. Lateral view of a finger showing osteophytes extending proximally at the DIP and PIP joints in a patient with osteoarthritis.

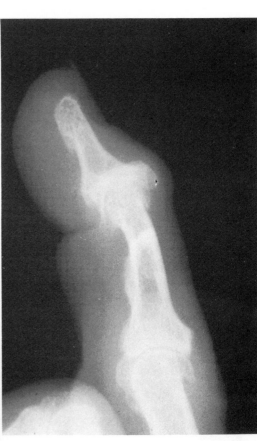

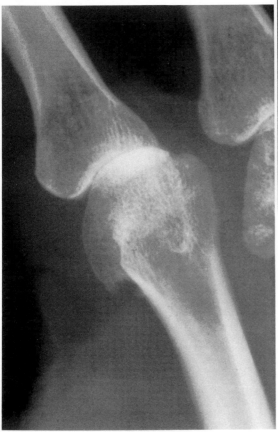

FIGURE 2–30. "Hook," or osteophyte, on the metacarpal head in a patient with CPPD.

DISTRIBUTION

Having evaluated the radiographic changes surrounding a specific joint, one must examine the distribution within the hand and wrist. Outlined below is the characteristic distribution with the digits.

DIP and PIP Involvement

Osteoarthritis—osteophytes without erosions
Erosive osteoarthritis—osteophytes and erosion
Psoriatic arthritis—erosion without osteophytes

MCP and PIP Involvement

Rheumatoid arthritis—erosions without new bone formation; spares the DIP's
Psoriatic arthritis, Reiter's disease, ankylosing spondylitis—erosions and new bone formation; will involve DIP's

MCP Involvement

Inflammatory arthropathies—erosions
CPPD (calcium pyrophosphate deposition disease)—osteophytes

Random Involvement

Gout

Carpal Involvement

The distribution in the wrist is also important in separating the arthropathies. The wrist is divided anatomically into specific compartments (Fig. 2–31), each of which is affected by different arthropathies. The inflammatory arthropathies involve all compartments causing erosions and joint space loss uniformly throughout the wrist (Fig. 2–32). New bone formation distinguishes the spondyloarthropathies from rheumatoid arthritis.

Osteoarthritis and erosive osteoarthritis involve only the first carpometacarpal joint and the greater multangular-navicular joint (Fig. 2–28). The presence of erosion differentiates one from the other. If osteoarthritic changes are present in the wrist in some other distribution, one must consider an etiology other than primary osteoarthritis. Often it may be a post-traumatic osteoarthritis (Fig. 2–33).

CPPD involves the radiocarpal compartment and often extends in a stair-step pattern to involve the capitate-lunate joint (Fig. 2–34). The changes in this distribution are those of osteoarthritis. Gout has a predilection for the carpometacarpal compartment, producing punched-out erosions with sclerotic borders (Fig. 2–35).

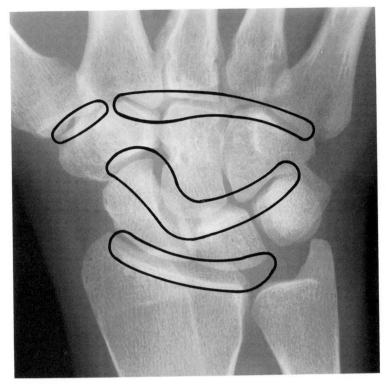

FIGURE 2–31. Normal wrist with outline of the different compartments: (1) the radiocarpal compartment, (2) the midcarpal compartment, (3) the common carpometacarpal compartment, and (4) the 1st carpometacarpal compartment. (From Brower AC: The radiologic approach to arthritis. Med Clin North Am 68:1593,1984.)

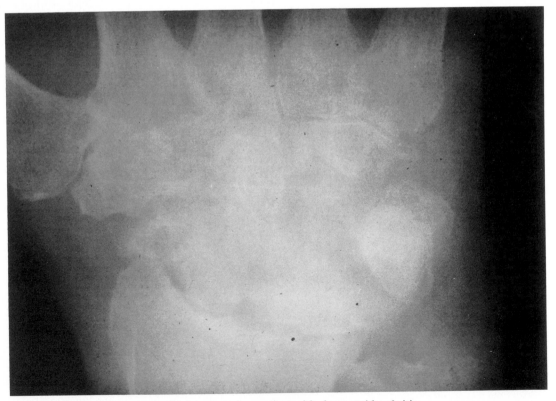

FIGURE 2–32. Pancarpal loss of joint spaces in a patient with rheumatoid arthritis.

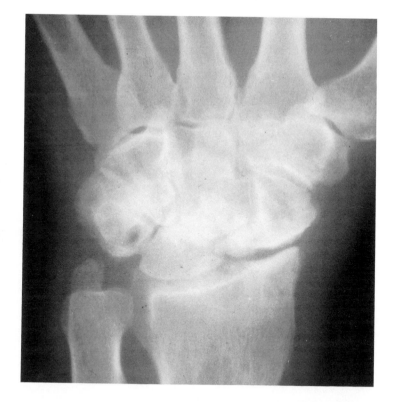

FIGURE 2–33. Narrowing of the capitate-lunate, the navicular-lunate, and the radiocarpal joints with subchondral sclerosis involving the capitate, lunate, navicula, and radius in a post-traumatic osteoarthritis. There is an old fracture of the navicular with osteonecrosis of the proximal fragment.

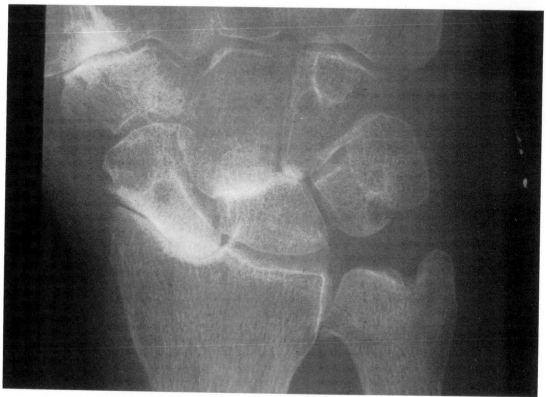

FIGURE 2–34. Narrowing of the radionavicular joint and the capitate-lunate joint with subchondral sclerosis surrounding these articulations in a patient with CPPD. (Courtesy of Dr. C. S. Resnik, University of Maryland.)

Seven radiographs are presented (Figs. 2–36 to 2–42), illustrating the common arthropathies involving the hand and summarizing all the individual features discussed in this chapter.

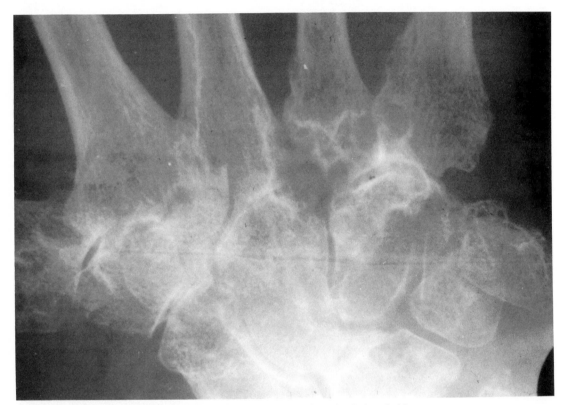

FIGURE 2–35. Erosive changes with sclerotic borders involving the 3rd and 4th carpo-metacarpal joint spaces in a patient with gout.

EARLY RHEUMATOID ARTHRITIS

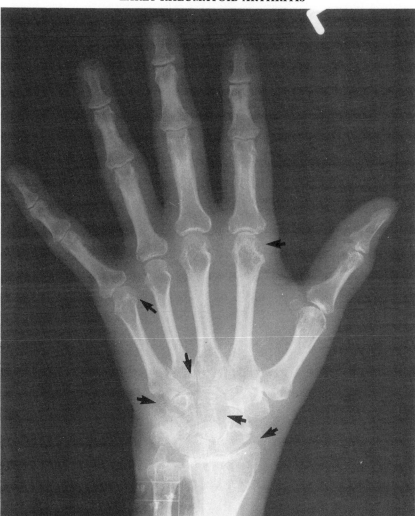

FIGURE 2–36

Soft tissue change:	Symmetrical swelling around PIP joints and wrist
Subluxations:	None
Mineralization:	Juxta-articular osteoporosis
Calcification:	None
Joint spaces:	Maintained
Erosions:	Early aggressive (arrows)
Bone production:	None
Distribution:	PIP's, MCP's, and pancarpal

LATE RHEUMATOID ARTHRITIS

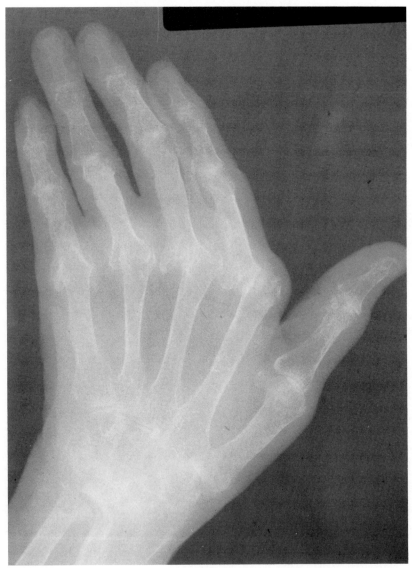

FIGURE 2–37

Soft tissue change:	Atrophy
Subluxations:	MCP joints (proximal phalanges subluxed ulnarly and palmarly)
Mineralization:	Diffuse osteoporosis
Calcification:	None
Joint spaces:	Uniform loss—PIP's, MCP's, and pancarpal
Erosions:	Large aggressive
Bone production:	None
Distribution:	PIP's, MCP's, and pancarpal

PSORIASIS

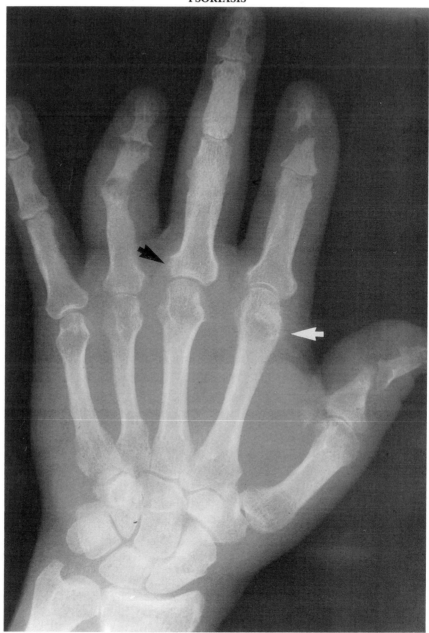

FIGURE 2–38

Soft tissue change:	Fusiform digit swelling—1st, 2nd, and 4th digits
Subluxations:	None
Mineralization:	Normal
Calcification:	None
Joint spaces:	Uniform loss—2nd and 4th MCP; destroyed 4th PIP, 1st IP, and 2nd DIP
Erosions:	Large, aggressive; pencil-in-cup erosion of IP joint of thumb
Bone production:	Solid periosteal new bone formation thickening 2nd and 3rd proximal and 3rd middle phalanges; fluffy new bone (arrows)
Distribution:	MCP's, PIP's, and DIP's, but in a ray distribution

(From Brower AC: The radiographic features of psoriatic arthritis. *In* Gerber L, Espinoza L (eds): Psoriatic Arthritis. Orlando, FL, Grune & Stratton, Inc, 1985, p 125.)

OSTEOARTHRITIS

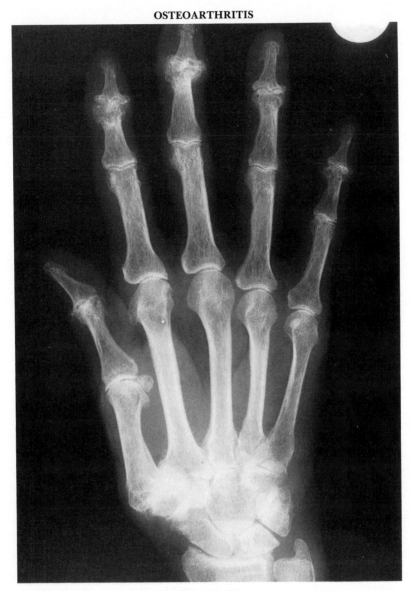

FIGURE 2–39

Soft tissue change:	Distortion around DIP's
Subluxations:	Laterally at 2nd and 3rd DIP
Mineralization:	Normal
Calcification:	None
Joint spaces:	Non-uniform loss—best seen at 2nd and 5th DIP's
Erosions:	None
Bone production:	Osteophytes at DIP's, 1st IP, and 1st and 2nd MCP; subchondral bone—greater multangular, distal navicula, and base of 1st metacarpal
Distribution:	DIP's, 1st IP and MCP; 1st C-MC joint and greater multangular–navicular joint

(From Brower AC: The radiologic approach to arthritis. Med Clin North Am 68:1593, 1984.)

EROSIVE OSTEOARTHRITIS

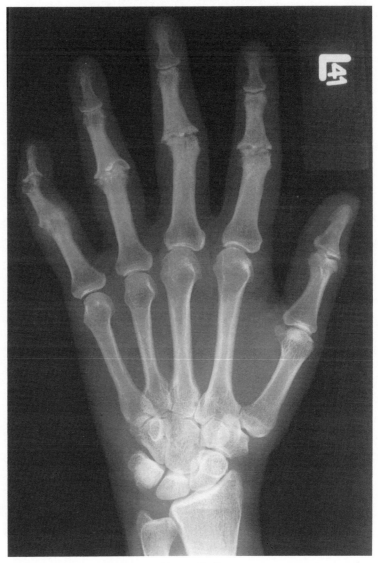

FIGURE 2–40

Soft tissue change:	None
Subluxations:	Laterally at 3rd and 4th PIP; flexion of 5th DIP
Mineralization:	Normal
Calcification:	None
Joint spaces:	Non-uniform loss—best seen at 3rd and 4th PIP
Erosions:	Central erosions—combined with osteophytes to produce "seagull" appearance
Bone production:	Osteophytes at PIP's and 5th DIP; subchondral sclerosis at 4th PIP
Distribution:	PIP's and 5th DIP

CPPD (CALCIUM PYROPHOSPHATE DEPOSITION) DISEASE

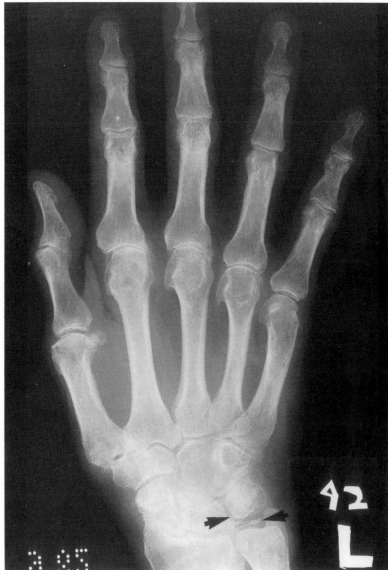

FIGURE 2–41

Soft tissue change:	None
Subluxations:	None
Mineralization:	Normal
Calcification:	Triangular cartilage (fibrous cartilage); between lunate and triquetrium (hyaline cartilage) (arrows)
Joint spaces:	Uniform loss of MCP's, radiocarpal, and capitate-lunate
Erosions:	None
Bone production:	Osteophytes at MCP joints; subchondral sclerosis in navicular, capitate, lunate
Distribution:	MCP's, radiocarpal, and capitate-lunate joints

(From Brower AC: The radiologic approach to arthritis. Med Clin North Am 68:1593, 1984.)

GOUT

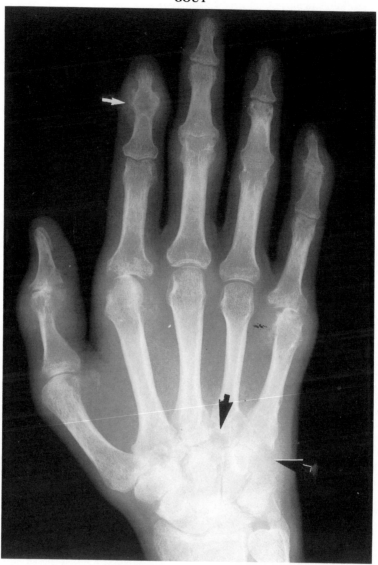

FIGURE 2–42

Soft tissue change:	Soft tissue mass around 2nd and 5th DIP, 1st IP, 2nd and 5th MCP
Subluxations:	Laterally at 2nd and 5th MCP
Mineralization:	Normal
Calcification:	In soft tissue masses—best seen at 2nd MCP
Joint spaces:	Maintained; non-uniform loss at 2nd and 5th MCP
Erosions:	Non-aggressive; 4th and 5th C-MC joints (large arrows), 2nd and 5th MCP joints, 1st IP joint, and 2nd DIP joint
Bone production:	Overhanging edge of cortex (small arrows)—5th metacarpal head and 2nd DIP joint
Distribution:	Carpometacarpal joint; randomly throughout fingers—2nd and 5th DIP, 1st IP, 2nd and 5th MCP

SUGGESTED READINGS

Bonavita JA, Dalinka MK, Schumacher HR: Hydroxyapatite deposition disease. Radiology 134:621–625, 1980.

Brower AC: The radiologic approach to arthritis. Med Clin North Am 68:1593–1607, 1984.

Kidd KL, Peter JB: Erosive osteoarthritis. Radiology 86:640, 1966.

Levine RB, Edeiken J: Arthritis: A radiologic approach. Applied Radiol July/Aug, 1985, pp 55–69.

Martel W: Diagnostic radiology in the rheumatic diseases. *In* Kelley WN, Harris ED, Ruddy S, et al. (eds): Textbook of Rheumatology. Philadelphia, W. B. Saunders Company, 1981.

Martel W: The overhanging margin of bone: A roentgenologic manifestation of gout. Radiology 91:755, 1968.

Martel W, Hayes JT, Duff IF: The pattern of bone erosion in the hand and wrist in rheumatoid arthritis. Radiology 84:204, 1965.

Martel W, Stuck KJ, Dworin AM, et al.: Erosive osteoarthritis and psoriatic arthritis: A radiologic comparison in the hand, wrist, and foot. AJR 134:125–135, 1980.

Norgaard F: Earliest roentgenological changes in polyarthritis of the rheumatoid type: Rheumatoid arthritis. Radiology 85:325, 1965.

Peter JB, Pearson CM, Marmar L: Erosive osteoarthritis of the hands. Arthritis Rheum 9:365, 1966.

Peterson CC, Silbiger ML: Reiter's syndrome and psoriatic arthritis: Their roentgen spectra and some interesting similarities. AJR 101:860–871, 1967.

Resnick D: Rheumatoid arthritis of the wrist: The compartmental approach. Med Radiogr Photogr 52:50–88, 1976.

Resnick D: The "target area" approach to articular disorders: A synopsis. *In* Resnick D, Niwayama G: Diagnosis of Bone and Joint Disorders with Emphasis on Articular Abnormalities. Philadelphia, W. B. Saunders Company, 1981, pp 3228–3255.

Resnik CS, Resnick D: Calcium pyrophosphate dihydrate crystal deposition disease. Curr Probl Diagn Radiol 11(6):40, 1982.

Sartoris DJ, Resnick D: Target area approach to arthritis of the small articulations. Contemp Diag Radiol 8:1–5, 1985.

chapter 3

APPROACH
TO THE HIP

The diagnosis of hip disease depends foremost on evaluation of the actual joint space. In some disorders the joint space is initially unaffected or even widened. Eventually, the femoral head migrates in one of three directions within the acetabulum, producing a specific pattern of joint space narrowing. The joint space narrows in either a superolateral direction, a medial direction, or an axial direction (Fig. 3–1).

SUPEROLATERAL MIGRATION

Superolateral migration of the femoral head within the acetabulum indicates a non-uniform loss of cartilage. The cartilage loss is confined to the upper outer portion of the articulation. This is usually secondary to change in the normal mechanical stress across the hip joint and is characteristic of osteoarthritis (Fig. 3–2). With this cartilage loss, subchondral bone, or reparative bone, as well as small osteophytes, is formed on the lateral aspect of the femoral head and acetabulum. Weight bearing is then shifted from the center of the femoral neck to the medial cortex of the femoral neck. As a result, new bone is laid down in apposition to the medial cortex. As the disease progresses, a large medial osteophyte forms on the femoral head to fill the lack of congruity between the acetabulum and the femoral head. Cystic changes are also part of osteoarthritis.

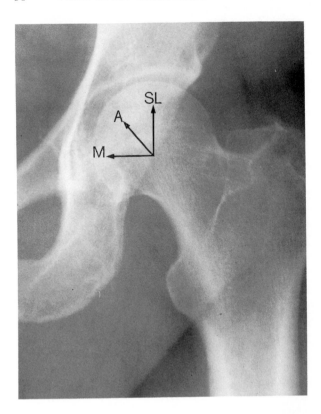

FIGURE 3–1. An AP view of a normal hip. Arrows show direction of femoral head migration with cartilage loss. Superolateral (SL), axial (A), medial (M). (From Brower AC: The radiologic approach to arthritis. Med Clin North Am 68:1593, 1984.)

FIGURE 3–2. AP view of the hip demonstrating changes of osteoarthritis: non-uniform loss of cartilage with superolateral narrowing, osteophyte formation, subchondral sclerosis, and new bone apposition along the medial cortex of the femoral neck (arrow).

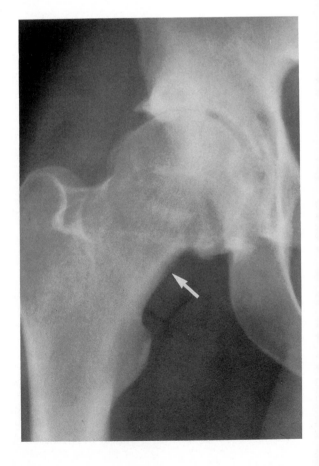

MEDIAL MIGRATION

Medial migration of the femoral head within the acetabulum is usually seen in patients who have sustained a fracture to the acetabulum (Fig. 3–3). This is accompanied by change in stress across the hip joint, causing non-uniform loss of cartilage medially. Osteoarthritic changes result.

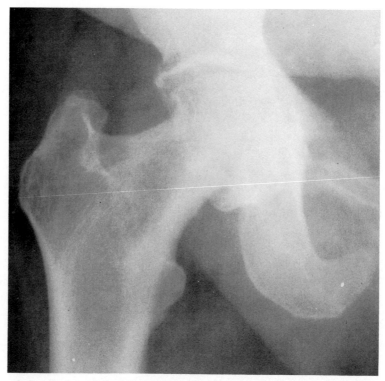

FIGURE 3–3. AP view of the hip showing fracture through the acetabulum. As a result, there is medial migration of the femoral head within the acetabulum with osteoarthritic changes.

AXIAL MIGRATION

Axial migration of the femoral head within the acetabulum, also called superomedial narrowing, indicates symmetrical uniform loss of cartilage. When the cartilage is affected uniformly, the earliest narrowing occurs along the axis of weight bearing or the axis of the femoral neck, as illustrated by a line drawn just superior to the fovea (Fig. 3–4). Axial migration is seen in any disease that involves the cartilage in a uniform fashion. This includes the inflammatory arthropathies, the crystalline arthropathies, and other arthropathies such as ochronosis and acromegaly. Upon observation of axial migration, one must evaluate the specific bone changes around the joint, such as mineralization, calcification, erosions, subchondral sclerosis, osteophyte formation, and cyst formation. The common arthropathies that produce axial migration are demonstrated, with emphasis on their differential changes.

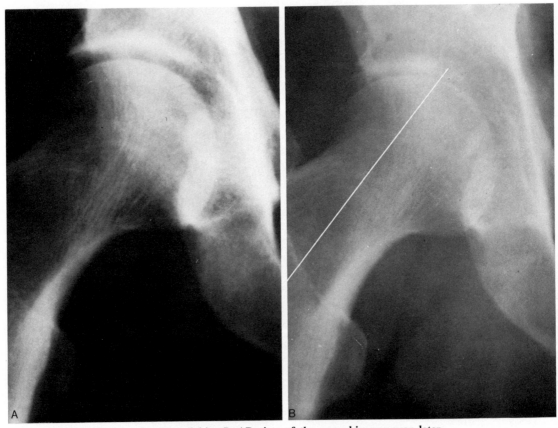

FIGURE 3–4. *A*, AP view of a normal hip. *B*, AP view of the same hip one year later demonstrating axial migration. The narrowest portion of the hip joint is along a line just superior to the fovea.

Rheumatoid Arthritis (Figs. 3–5 and 3–6)

This is a bilateral symmetrical disease progressing from axial migration to acetabuli protrusio (Fig. 3–5). The bony structures are osteoporotic. There is little if any subchondral bone sclerosis. There is no osteophyte formation and no bone apposition along the inner aspect of the femoral neck. Erosions, when present, are relatively small. Synovial cysts may or may not be present. The hallmark is bilateral symmetrical axial migration with osteoporosis and lack of any evidence of bone repair (Fig. 3–6).

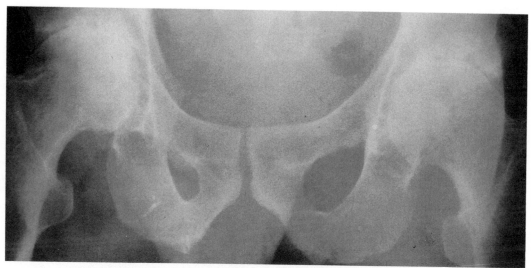

FIGURE 3–5. AP view of the pelvis showing bilateral symmetrical uniform narrowing of the hip joints. Both heads have moved in an axial direction. There is generalized osteoporosis. There is no evidence of osteophyte formation or bone apposition along the inner aspect of the femoral neck. There is little if any subchondral bone repair.

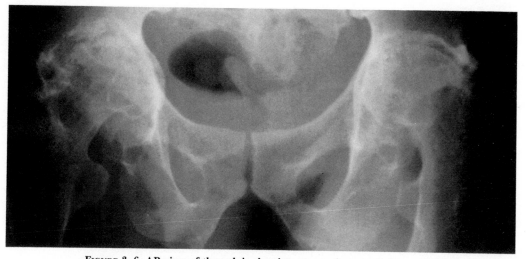

FIGURE 3–6. AP view of the pelvis showing severe changes of rheumatoid arthritis. There is bilateral acetabuli protrusio. Note that the axial migration is actually superomedial. There is severe osteoporosis and lack of significant bone repair.

Ankylosing Spondylitis (Figs. 3–7 and 3–8)

Ankylosing spondylitis causes bilateral symmetrical axial migration of both hips, without producing the severe acetabuli protrusio seen in rheumatoid arthritis. At first mineralization is maintained, and a cuff of osteophytes is seen at the junction of the femoral head and neck along with osteophytes at the superior and inferior borders of the acetabulum (Fig. 3–7). Unlike rheumatoid arthritis, ankylosing spondylitis is an ossifying disease. Erosive or cystic changes may not play a significant role in the changes in the hip. Instead the hip tends to progress to true bone ankylosis. The ankylosed femoral head tends to be almost normal in contour. Once ankylosis takes place, the surrounding bone structures become osteoporotic (Fig. 3–8).

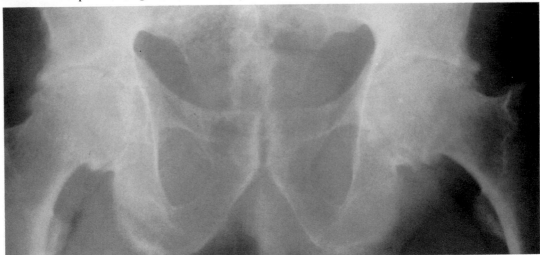

FIGURE 3–7. AP view of the pelvis in a patient with ankylosing spondylitis. There is uniform loss of the cartilage with axial migration of both femoral heads. There is a cuff of osteophytes formed at the junction of the head and neck bilaterally. There are also osteophytes found on the superior and inferior aspects of the acetabulum. Note the ankylosis of the SI joints and the whiskering of the ischial tuberosities.

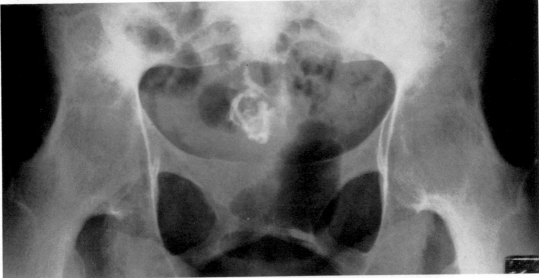

FIGURE 3–8. AP view of the pelvis in a patient with late-stage ankylosing spondylitis. There is total ankylosis of the SI joints, the hip joints, and the pubic symphysis. Note that through the ankylosis the contour of the femoral head is fairly well maintained. The bony structures are osteoporotic.

Calcium Pyrophosphate Dihydrate (CPPD) Crystal Deposition Disease (Figs. 3–9 and 3–10)

In CPPD crystal deposition disease both hips are involved either symmetrically or, more commonly, asymmetrically. Before axial migration occurs, one may observe calcification of the articular cartilage (Fig. 3–9). The axial migration rarely progresses to the extensive acetabuli protrusio seen in rheumatoid arthritis. Unlike the inflammatory arthropathies, there is degeneration rather than active destruction of the cartilage. Therefore, the process is more indolent, and secondary osteoarthritic changes develop in the surrounding bones. Subchondral sclerosis, osteophyte formation, and cystic changes are seen (Fig. 3–10). The osteophytes formed tend to be smaller than those formed in osteoarthritis. Since there is no incongruity between the femoral head and the acetabulum, the large medial osteophyte seen in mechanical osteoarthritis is not seen in CPPD arthropathy. Cyst formation is more prevalent in CPPD arthropathy than in mechanical osteoarthritis. Severe CPPD arthropathy of the hip may resemble the changes of a neuropathic hip with no semblance of a joint space, massive bone repair, excessive osteophytosis, and bone debris.

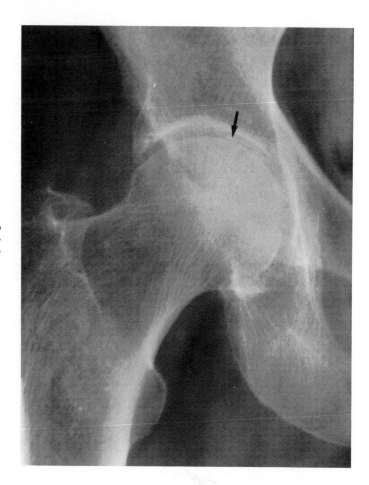

FIGURE 3–9. An AP view of the hip demonstrating presence of chondro-calcinosis (arrow) and early axial migration of the head within the joint.

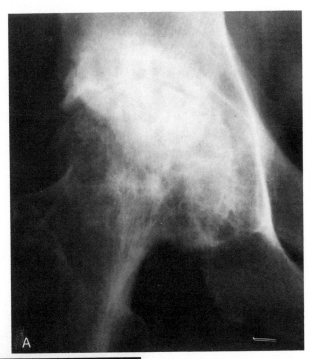

FIGURE 3–10. *A*, AP view of the hip in a patient with CPPD arthropathy. There is uniform loss of cartilage with axial migration present. There is significant subchondral bone repair and cyst formation. Osteophytes are also present. *B*, Specimen radiograph of the femoral head pictured in *A*. The cyst and reparative bone are well seen. Chondrocalcinosis is present in the remaining fragment of cartilage (arrow).

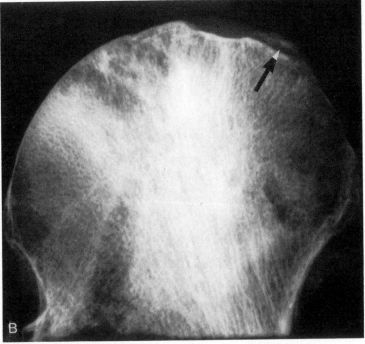

Septic Arthritis (Figs. 3–11 and 3–12)

Although the literature describes initial widening of a joint space with septic arthritis, usually we first see uniform narrowing of the joint space. The adjacent bony structures are osteoporotic. The diagnosis is clear when absence of the white cortical line along an extensive portion of the femoral head is observed (Fig. 3–11). Normally, as the entire white cortical line is lost and the underlying bone is destroyed, secondary reparative bone will be laid down behind the destruction. However, with an aggressive septic arthritis and resultant osteomyelitis, the entire femoral head and acetabulum can be destroyed without any evidence of repair (Fig. 3–12).

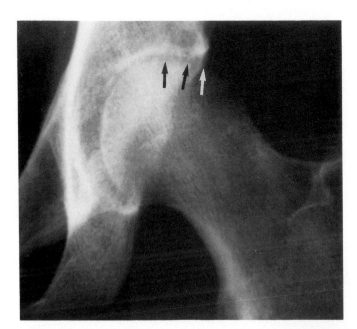

FIGURE 3–11. AP view of the hip with septic arthritis. There is axial migration of the femoral head within the acetabulum. There is significant loss of the white cortical line along the superolateral aspect of the femoral head (arrows).

FIGURE 3–12. AP view of the hip with septic arthritis going on to osteomyelitis. There has been total destruction of the femoral head and a large portion of the neck. There is considerable destruction of the acetabulum as well. Bone debris is seen within the joint space. This might be mistaken for a neuropathic hip except that the margin of destruction is extremely irregular and there is adjacent osteoporosis.

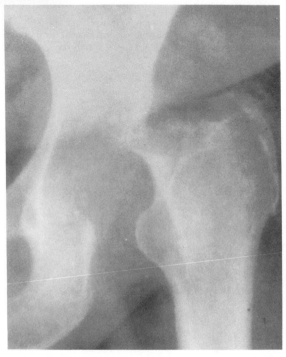

Axial migration of the femoral head within the acetabulum may take place secondary to underlying bone disease rather than as primary disease of the cartilage (Fig. 3–13). The two most common bone diseases that cause this are Paget's disease and renal osteodystrophy. In both instances, the underlying bone cannot absorb the normal stress applied to the acetabular area, and the acetabulum protrudes inward with weight bearing. The hip follows to maintain continuity within the acetabulum. Secondary degenerative changes commonly develop.

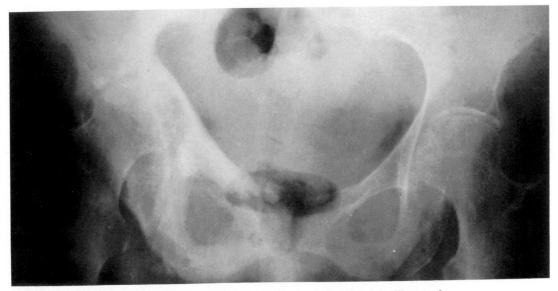

FIGURE 3–13. AP view of the pelvis with Paget's disease involving the right ilium and ischium. The right hip has moved in an axial direction, with a resultant protrusion of the acetabulum secondary to the Paget's disease.

NORMAL JOINT SPACE

There are four common disorders involving the hip joint which will not cause loss of the actual joint until late in the disease. These are osteonecrosis of the femoral head, synovial osteochondromatosis, pigmented villonodular synovitis, and tuberculosis.

Osteonecrosis (Figs. 3–14 and 3–16)

Osteonecrosis of the femoral head, no matter what the etiology, is a disorder of the femoral head. Only after the anatomical contour of the femoral head has been distorted and the overlying cartilage secondarily disrupted will the joint become involved with secondary osteoarthritis. In the earlier stages of osteonecrosis, the joint space is completely maintained and the acetabulum is completely normal. The first radiographic changes in the femoral head will be seen as smudginess of the normal trabecular pattern (Fig. 3–14). (The role of scintigraphy and MRI is discussed in Chapter 1.) As repair occurs, lytic and sclerotic areas will be seen throughout the femoral head. The subchondral crescent-shaped lucency, seen best with the frogleg lateral view, is a rather late stage of necrosis and indicates impending collapse of the femoral head and the overlying cartilage (Fig. 3–15). Once this collapse has occurred, secondary osteoarthritic changes will develop (Fig. 3–16). However, one can distinguish late-stage osteonecrosis with secondary osteoarthritis from late-stage biomechanical osteoarthritis; in the late stages of osteonecrosis and secondary osteoarthritis, the radiographic changes in the femoral head are far more extensive than those in the acetabulum, whereas in late-stage mechanical osteoarthritis, the bone changes are equally distributed between the acetabulum and the femoral head.

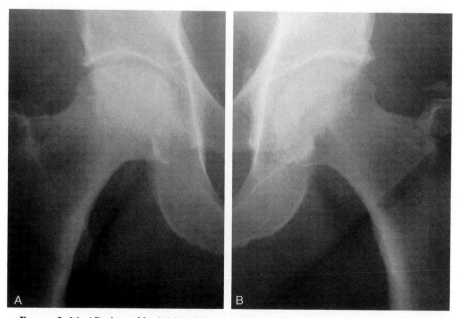

FIGURE 3–14. AP view of both hips demonstrating a normal left hip (*B*) and osteonecrosis of the right femoral head (*A*). Note that the joint space is maintained. The acetabulum is within normal limits. The trabecular pattern of the right femoral head has become smudgy as compared to the trabecular pattern of the left femoral head.

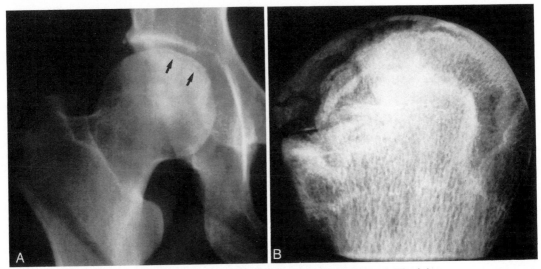

FIGURE 3–15. *A*, AP view of the hip showing osteonecrosis of the femoral head. The joint space is maintained. The acetabulum is within normal limits. There are smudginess of the trabecular pattern and a subchondral lucency (arrows), indicating impending collapse. *B*, Specimen radiograph of a femoral head with osteonecrosis. Subchondral lucency and collapse beneath are well demonstrated.

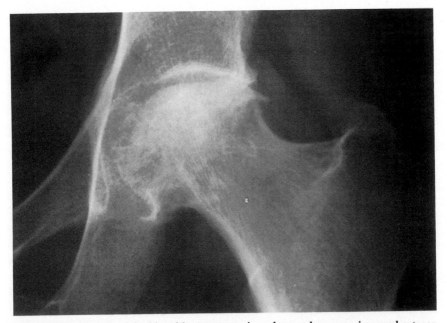

FIGURE 3–16. AP view of the hip with osteonecrosis and secondary superimposed osteoarthritic changes. Note that most of the radiographic abnormalities are present in the femoral head rather than in the acetabulum. However, the joint space is now lost in the superolateral aspect.

Synovial Chondromatosis (Figs. 3–17 and 3–18)

There is no difficulty in making this diagnosis radiographically if the chondroid bodies are ossified sufficiently to be recognized (Fig. 3–17). If the bodies are not ossified, one must rely on other radiographic signs to make the diagnosis. The joint space is usually normal but may actually be widened or, late in the disease, narrowed. Osteoporosis of the bony structures may be present. The best radiographic sign is scalloping defects along the neck of the femur, usually most pronounced at the junction of the head and the neck (Fig. 3–18). Arthrography is the definitive study.

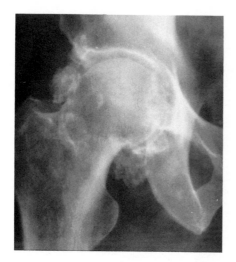

FIGURE 3–17. AP view of the hip with synovial osteochondromatosis. The joint space is maintained. The joint capsule is filled with ossified chondroid bodies.

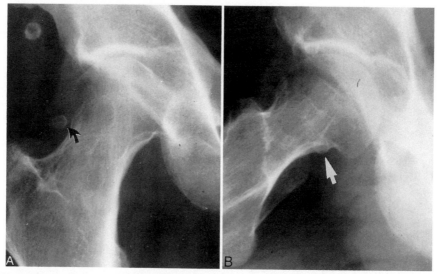

FIGURE 3–18. Synovial osteochondromatosis of the hip. *A,* AP view demonstrates a normal joint space. There is surrounding osteoporosis. There are scalloped defects on the femoral neck, one producing a sharp angle to the head as it joins the neck inferiorly. There are two calcific densities present. The superior one is an injection granuloma. The inferior one (arrow) is within the joint, as proved by the frogleg view. *B,* The frogleg view of the same hip again shows the inferior calcific density (arrow) to be within the hip joint, representing an ossified synovial osteochondroma. Note the scalloped defects of the femoral neck, especially at the junction of the head and neck. (Courtesy of Dr. H. Genant, University of California, San Francisco.)

Pigmented Villonodular Synovitis (Fig. 3–19)

The radiographic changes are somewhat similar to those of synovial osteochondromatosis. The joint space may be normal, slightly widened, or, in the late stages, narrowed. Osteoporosis may or may not be present. Well-defined cysts are seen on both sides of the joint. Scalloping defects may be seen in the femoral neck, especially at the junction of the femoral head and neck. There is little evidence of bone repair or osteophyte formation. The patient's age and the single joint involvement help to confirm the diagnosis, and the cystic changes help to distinguish it from synovial osteochondromatosis. Tuberculosis can present a similar appearance.

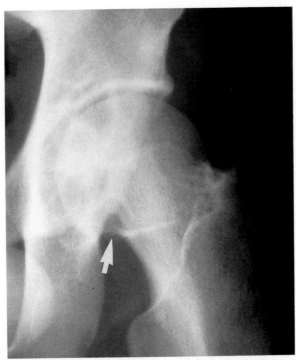

FIGURE 3–19. AP view of the hip in a patient with pigmented villonodular synovitis. The hip joint is maintained. There is normal mineralization present. There are cystic changes in the acetabulum as well as in the femoral head. The scalloping defect seen at the junction of the femoral head with the neck (arrow) demonstrates that the femoral head and neck are involved as well as the acetabulum.

SUGGESTED READINGS

Bullough P, Goodfellow J, O'Conner J: Relationship between degenerative changes and load-bearing in human hip. J Bone Joint Surg 55B:746–758, 1973.

Butt WP: Radiology of the infected joint. Clin Orthop Rel Res 96:136, 1973.

Dwosh IL, Resnick D, Becker MA: Hip involvement in ankylosing spondylitis. Arthritis Rheum 19:683, 1976.

Goldman AB, Bullough P, Kammerman S, Ambos M: Osteitis deformans of the hip joint. AJR 128:601–606, 1977.

Murray R: Aetiology of primary osteoarthritis of the hip. Br J Radiol 38:810–824, 1965.

Resnick D: Patterns of femoral head migration in osteoarthritis of the hip: Roentgenographic-pathologic correlation and comparison with rheumatoid arthritis. AJR 124:62–74, 1975.

Resnick D: Radiographic approach to hip disease. Radiolog 1(3):27–44, 1978.

Resnick D, Niwayama G, Goergen TG, et al.: Clinical, radiographic and pathologic abnormalities in calcium pyrophosphate dihydrate deposition disease (CPPD): Pseudogout. Radiology 122:1–15, 1977.

Scott PM: Bone lesions in pigmented villonodular synovitis. J Bone Joint Surg 50B:306–311, 1968.

Sweet DE, Madewell JE: Pathogenesis of osteonecrosis. In Resnick D, Niwayama G (eds): Diagnosis of Bone and Joint Disorders, Vol 3. Philadelphia, W. B. Saunders Company, 1981.

Zimmerman C, Sayegh V: Roentgen manifestations of synovial osteochondromatosis. AJR 83:680, 1960.

chapter 4

APPROACH
TO THE KNEE

As in the hip, the diagnosis of a disorder of the knee depends foremost on the evaluation of true joint space involvement. This evaluation is made most accurately through an AP standing view of the knee and a flexed lateral view (see Chapter 1). The joint consists of three compartments: the medial tibiofemoral compartment, the lateral tibiofemoral compartment, and the patellofemoral compartment. The various arthropathies are characterized by the manner in which they affect these compartments. They separate into the following categories: those that affect all three compartments, those that preferentially involve a specific compartment, and those that initially do not involve any compartment.

TOTAL COMPARTMENT INVOLVEMENT

Total compartment narrowing indicates that all three compartments of the knee are involved in a uniform manner. This implies a primary abnormality of the underlying cartilage leading to loss. This loss may be caused either by aggressive destruction from inflammation or by slow degeneration secondary to deposition of foreign substance into the cartilage. The latter is seen in the late phases of the crystalline arthropathies, ochronosis, acromegaly, and the neuropathic joint. The early phases of these arthropathies are discussed elsewhere in this chapter. However, once there is uniform loss of the cartilage, osteoarthritic changes are seen in the adjacent tibia, femur, and patella. Although it is difficult to distinguish one arthropathy from another in this osteoarthritic phase of disease, the uniform involvement of all compartments will separate these arthropathies from common mechanical osteoarthritis.

The arthropathies that produce total compartment involvement by aggressive destruction are the inflammatory arthropathies. Each has specific radiographic characteristics that distinguish it from the others.

Rheumatoid Arthritis (Figs. 4–1 and 4–2)

Rheumatoid arthritis is a bilateral symmetrical disease producing uniform loss of all compartments of the knee and generalized osteoporosis. Despite the fact that the knee is a weight-bearing joint, there is little evidence of bone repair or osteophyte formation in response to the cartilage loss (Fig. 4–1). Erosive changes may be present but are not a prominent part of the radiographic picture. Large synovial cysts may be present. A cyst may become so large as to resemble a bone neoplasm (Fig. 4–2). However, observation of uniform loss of joint space as well as smaller cysts in the adjacent bone should prevent an erroneous diagnosis. Occasionally there will be preferential narrowing of the lateral compartment. However, the relative lack of bone response to this loss should direct one away from the diagnosis of a mechanical osteoarthritis and indicate the correct diagnosis of rheumatoid arthritis.

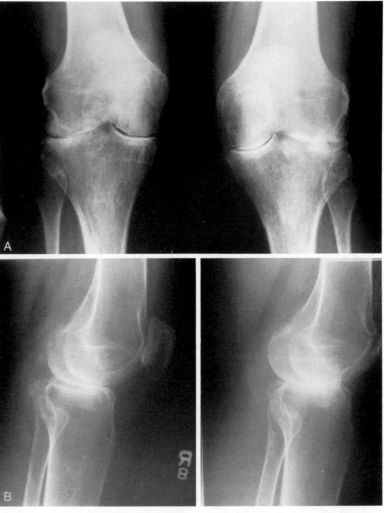

FIGURE 4–1. *A*, AP standing view of both knees and (*B*) lateral view of both knees in a patient with rheumatoid arthritis. There is loss of cartilage in all compartments. There is generalized osteoporosis with little to no evidence of bone repair. (*A* from Kantor S, Brower AC: Radiographic assessment. *In* Rothermich N, Whisler R: Rheumatoid Arthritis, Orlando, FL, Grune & Stratton, Inc, 1985, p 57.)

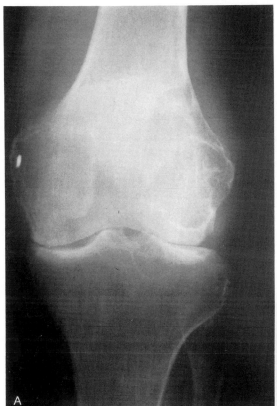

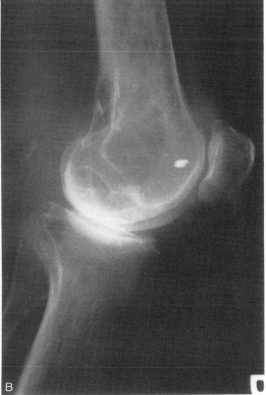

FIGURE 4–2. *A*, AP and (*B*) lateral views of the knee in a patient with rheumatoid arthritis. The large synovial cyst involves the lateral femoral condyle and resembles a giant cell tumor. However, there is narrowing of all compartments, generalized osteoporosis, and a synovial cyst involving the adjacent tibial plateau. (From Kantor S, Brower AC: Radiographic assessment. *In* Rothermich N, Whisler R: Rheumatoid Arthritis, Orlando, FL, Grune & Stratton, Inc, 1985, p. 57.)

Psoriatic Arthritis or Reiter's Disease (Fig. 4–3)

Psoriatic arthritis and Reiter's disease present similar radiographic changes. Both are a bilateral but asymmetrical disease, involving one knee more than the other or involving one portion of the knee more than another. Unlike rheumatoid arthritis, bone mineralization is maintained. Also unlike rheumatoid arthritis, there is usually evidence of bone proliferation in the form of bone excrescences at ligamentous and tendinous attachments or a periostitis.

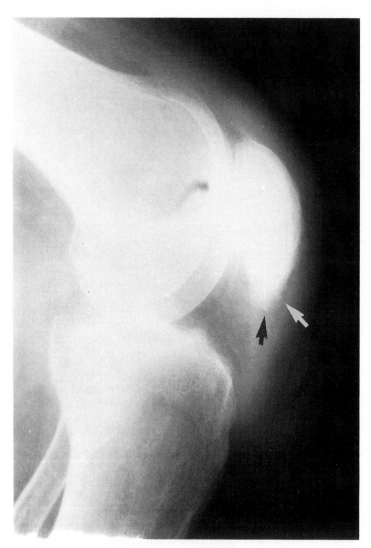

FIGURE 4–3. Lateral view of the knee in psoriatic arthritis. There is bone proliferation on the anterior inferior surface of the patella (arrows). (From Brower AC: The radiographic features of psoriatic arthritis. *In* Gerber L, Espinoza L (eds): Psoriatic Arthritis. Orlando, FL, Grune & Stratton, Inc, 1985, p 125.)

Ankylosing Spondylitis (Fig. 4–4)

Knee involvement in ankylosing spondylitis is uncommon. However, when knee involvement is present, ankylosis is the predominant part of the radiographic picture. Early in the disease process, small erosions with adjacent bone sclerosis will be present. However, in a relatively short period of time the joint will ankylose, leaving normal contour to the ghost joint margins.

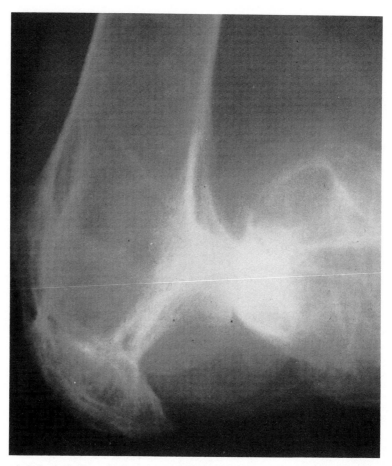

FIGURE 4–4. Lateral view of a knee in a patient with long-standing ankylosing spondylitis. The knee is ankylosed in a flexed position. The normal contours of the knee are seen through the ankylosis.

Juvenile Chronic Arthritis (Fig. 4–5)

Most frequently this presents as unilateral disease, but with total compartment involvement of the affected knee. The most prominent feature is overgrowth of the femoral and tibial epiphyses as well as overgrowth of the patella; with the overgrowth of the femoral condyles, the intracondylar notch appears widened. Since the cartilage is thicker in the child than in the adult, erosive disease and cyst formation, if present, are late manifestations. It may be difficult to distinguish these radiographic changes from those produced in hemophilia.

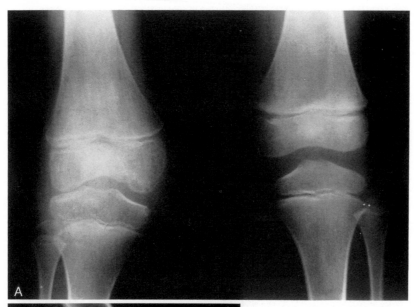

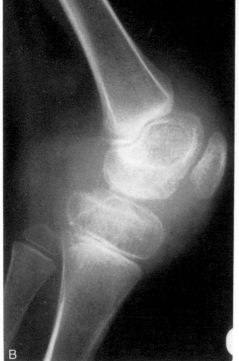

FIGURE 4–5. *A,* AP standing view of both knees in a patient with juvenile rheumatoid arthritis. The right leg is longer than the left leg. There is overgrowth of the femoral and tibial epiphyses in the right knee. There are uniform loss of cartilage and small erosive changes on the medial femoral condyle. *B,* Lateral view of the right knee. A large effusion is present. There is overgrowth of the femoral and tibial epiphyses. There is also overgrowth of the patella. The patella is elongated in configuration compared to the square configuration seen in the hemophilic knee (Fig. 4–7).

Hemophilia (Fig. 4–6) also produces overgrowth of the epiphyses and patella and widening of the intracondylar notch. There tends to be more cyst formation in the hemophilic knee, secondary to intraosseous bleeding, than in the juvenile rheumatoid knee. It has also been observed that the overgrown patella becomes square in hemophilia (Fig. 4–7) and elongated in the inflammatory arthropathy of childhood.

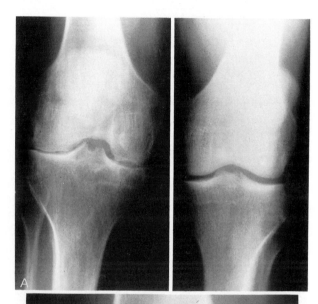

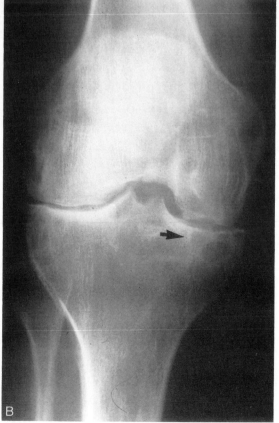

FIGURE 4–6. *A*, AP standing view of both knees in a patient with hemophilia. The right knee is involved while the left knee is spared. *B*, Close-up AP view of the right knee. There is overgrowth of the femoral and tibial epiphyses with widening of the intercondylar notch. There is uniform loss of the joint space visualized. A cyst is seen in the medial tibial plateau (arrow).

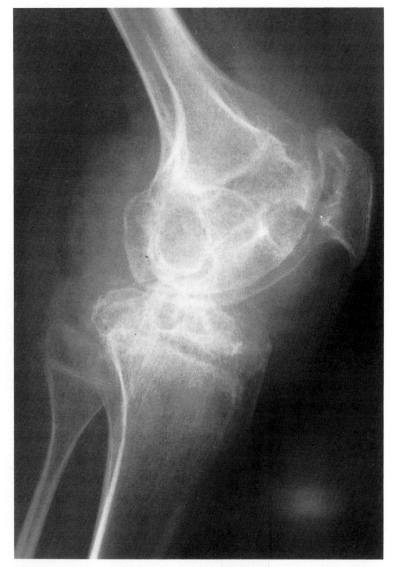

FIGURE 4–7. Lateral view of the knee in a patient with hemophilia. Synovial proliferation is seen. There is overgrowth of the femoral and tibial epiphyses as well as the patella, which is square in shape. Multiple cysts are seen in the epiphyses and patella.

Septic Arthritis (Figs. 4–8 and 4–9)

Septic arthritis presents as unilateral involvement. In aggressive disease there will be evidence of effusion, uniform cartilage loss, juxta-articular osteoporosis, and diagnostic loss of the white cortical line (Fig. 4–8). As bone is destroyed, attempts at repair are usually made behind the destruction. In more indolent disease, such as tuberculous or fungal disease, there may be relative preservation of the joint space and erosions at the margins of the joint (Fig. 4–9). In childhood, an indolent infection may have a radiographic appearance similar to that of juvenile chronic arthritis.

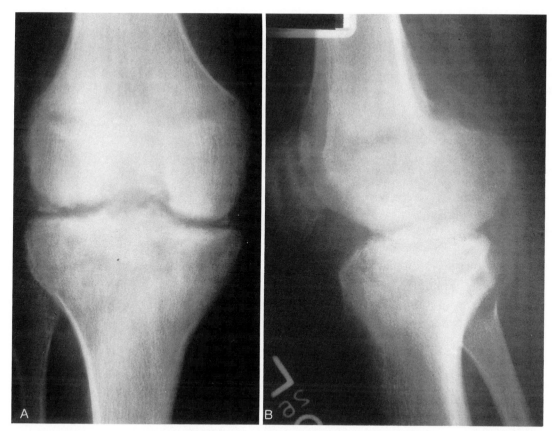

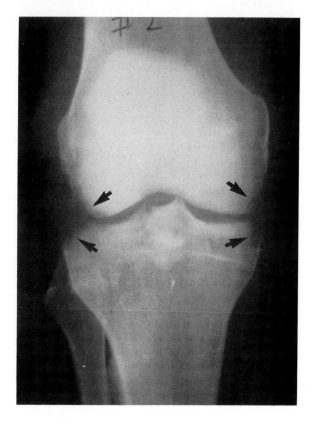

FIGURE 4–8. AP (*A*) and lateral (*B*) views of a knee with septic arthritis. There is cartilage loss in all compartments of the knee. There is loss of the white cortical line best seen on the AP view. There is evidence of bone repair. (From Resnick D, Niwayama G: Osteomyelitis, septic arthritis and soft tissue infection: The organisms. *In* Diagnosis of Bone and Joint Disorders. Vol. 2. Philadelphia, W. B. Saunders Company, 1981.)

FIGURE 4–9. AP view of a knee with tuberculous arthritis. The joint space appears to be preserved. Erosions are present at the margins of the joint (arrows).

PREFERENTIAL COMPARTMENT LOSS

Two common arthropathies involve specific compartments in the knee joint, and knowledge of this specific compartment involvement helps the radiologist to make the correct diagnosis. These two arthropathies are (1) primary osteoarthritis and (2) calcium pyrophosphate dihydrate (CPPD) crystal deposition disease.

Osteoarthritis (Fig. 4–10)

Osteoarthritis of the knee is the most common arthropathy of the knee. It develops from change in the normal mechanisms of weight bearing across the knee joint. It is seen most commonly in patients with past significant trauma and in obese females. The normal standing knee shows slight valgus angulation. Most osteoarthritic knees stand in varus. There is preferential loss of the medial tibiofemoral compartment and associated loss of the patellofemoral compartment. As the cartilage is lost, there is evidence of bone repair with subchondral sclerosis and osteophyte formation. Cystic changes are part of the radiographic picture. Occasionally the lateral tibiofemoral compartment shows preferential loss, and an extreme valgus deformity is demonstrated on standing views. The patellofemoral compartment is not as commonly affected with lateral compartment involvement as with medial compartment involvement.

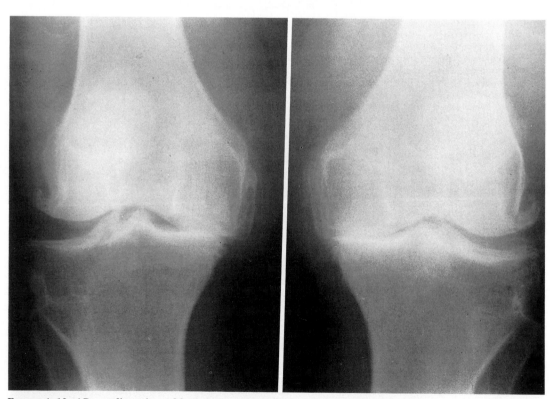

FIGURE 4–10. AP standing view of both knees in a patient with osteoarthritis. There is preferential loss of the medial tibiofemoral compartment. There is subchondral bone formation and osteophyte formation.

When osteoarthritic changes become exuberant one must consider the possibility of a **neuropathic joint** (Fig. 4–11). The early radiographic changes in the neuropathic knee are massive recurrent effusions, subluxations, pathological fracture, and bone debris within the joint. As the process progresses, there is complete dissolution of the joint space, exuberant bone formation or eburnation, massive osteophytosis, and bone fragmentation.

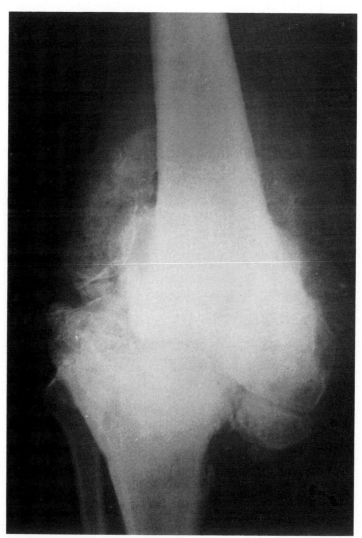

FIGURE 4–11. AP view of a neuropathic knee. There are joint dissolution, subluxation, eburnation, fragmentation, and osseous debris. (From Brower AC, Allman RM: The neuropathic joint—A neurovascular bone disorder. Radiol Clin North Am 19:571–580, 1981.)

Calcium Pyrophosphate Dihydrate (CPPD) Crystal Deposition Disease (Figs. 4–12 and 4–13)

This is the second most common arthropathy of the knee, and it is seen predominantly in the elderly. There is preferential involvement of the patellofemoral joint space (Fig. 4–12). The narrowing of this joint space is accompanied by subchondral bone sclerosis and osteophyte formation on the posterior aspect of the patella and the anterior aspect of the femoral condyles. The narrowing may be so severe as to allow the motion of the patella to create a scalloped defect in the femur superior to the location of the patella in the flexed view. The defect is actually where the patella abuts the femur in extension. This radiographic change may be present even though the medial and lateral tibiofemoral compartments are unaffected. However, usually one can identify chondrocalcinosis in the maintained compartments. In some patients, all compartments of the knee may be involved with cartilage loss and osteoarthritic changes. In such patients, the presence of chondrocalcinosis may be impossible to identify. It is the one arthropathy in which the osteoarthritic changes may become so exuberant as to resemble those of a neuropathic knee (Fig. 4–13).

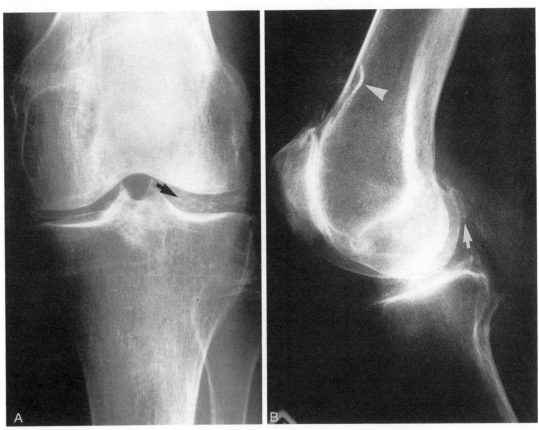

FIGURE 4–12. AP (*A*) and lateral (*B*) views of a knee in a patient with CPPD arthropathy. The medial and lateral tibiofemoral compartments are maintained, and chondrocalcinosis is identified (arrows). There is total loss of the patellofemoral joint space with adjacent subchondral new bone formation. A scalloped defect is seen in the femur (arrowhead) which is created by the patella as it abuts the femur when the knee is in extension. (From Brower AC: The radiologic approach to arthritis. Med Clin North Am 68:1593, 1984.)

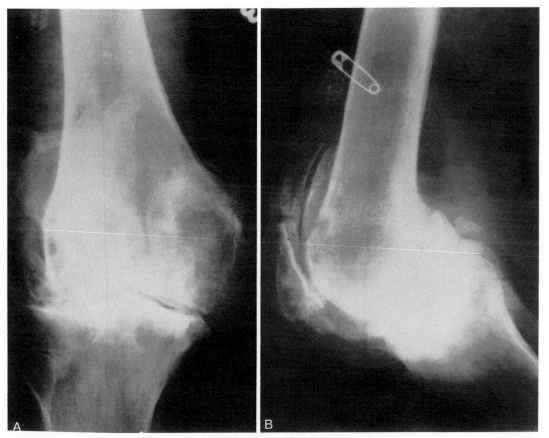

FIGURE 4–13. AP (*A*) lateral (*B*) views of a knee in a patient with CPPD arthropathy. There is extensive eburnation, massive osteophytosis, fragmentation, and osseous debris. The appearance suggests a neuropathic knee.

NORMAL JOINT SPACE

As in the hip, there are four common disorders of the knee joint that do not cause actual loss of the joint until late in the disease. These are osteonecrosis, osteochondritis dissecans, synovial osteochondromatosis, and pigmented villonodular synovitis.

Osteonecrosis (Figs. 4–14 to 4–16)

Osteonecrosis of the femoral condyle has long been recognized as occurring in certain diseases, such as systemic lupus erythematosus (SLE), and as a complication of steroid therapy. Only recently has it been recognized as a relatively common idiopathic disorder in the elderly. Since it is a disease process of the femoral condyle, initially the joint itself is not affected. First detection of this disorder is usually made through bone scintigraphy. Radiographically one initially sees ill-defined areas of lucency and bone repair in the involved condyle (Fig. 4–14). A subchondral lucency and displacement of the cortical fragment inward are pathognomonic of osteonecrosis (Fig. 4–15). As the disease progresses, there is marked deformity to the femoral condyle (Fig. 4–16); only in the late phases does secondary osteoarthritis develop. Although either condyle may be affected, it occurs more commonly in the medial condyle.

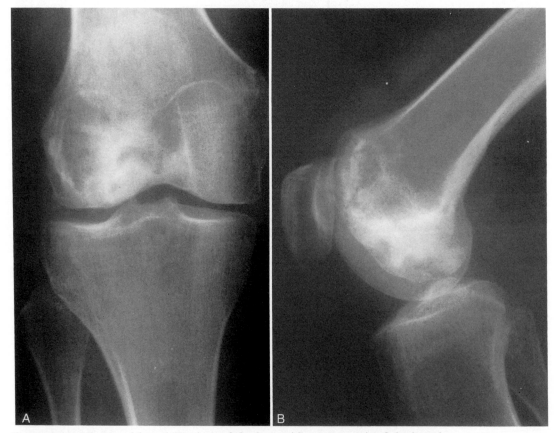

FIGURE 4–14. AP (*A*) and lateral (*B*) views of the knee with osteonecrosis of the lateral femoral condyle. The joint space is maintained. The radiographic abnormalities are limited to the lateral femoral condyle and are identified as ill-defined areas of lucency and bone repair.

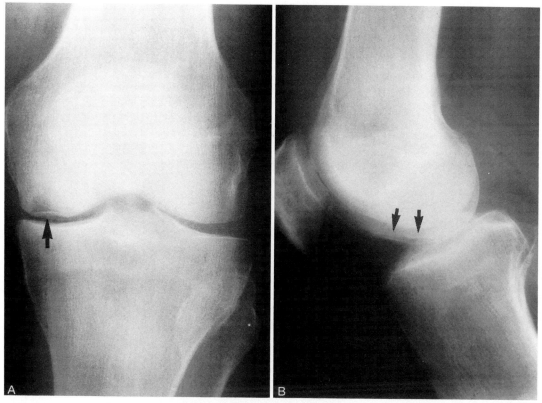

FIGURE 4–15. AP (*A*) and lateral (*B*) views of the knee with early osteonecrosis involving the medial femoral condyle. The subchondral lucency and displacement of the cortical fragment inward (arrows) are pathognomonic radiological signs of osteonecrosis.

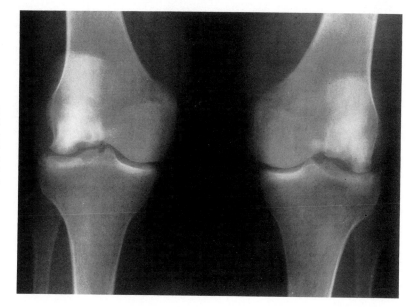

FIGURE 4–16. AP standing view of the knees in a patient with SLE. Both lateral condyles are markedly deformed secondary to osteonecrosis. The lateral tibiofemoral compartments are minimally narrowed.

Osteochondritis Dissecans (Fig. 4–17)

This is a disorder of the relatively young. It is an osteochondral fragment and defect seen in the lateral anterior aspect of the medial femoral condyle. It is a result of chronic repetitive trauma to an area of normal irregular ossification during growth. The bone part of the fragment may be identified within the defect or free within the joint; also, it may not be visualized at all owing to resorption. However, the cartilage part of the fragment is present but may have to be imaged by arthrography. The defect in the femoral condyle has a relatively well-defined sclerotic border. This definition and location distinguish osteochondritis dissecans from osteonecrosis of the femoral condyle.

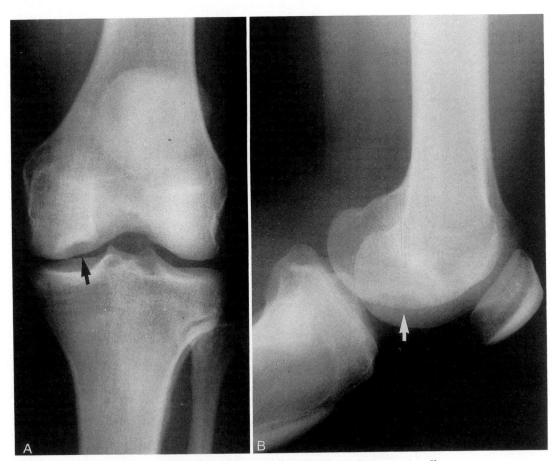

FIGURE 4–17. AP (*A*) and lateral (*B*) views of a knee with osteochondritis dissecans. A well-defined defect with a sclerotic border is seen in the lateral anterior aspect of the medial condyle (arrows). The osteochondral fragment is not identified. The ossific portion has been resorbed. An arthrogram would identify the cartilage portion.

Synovial Osteochondromatosis (Fig. 4–18)

As with the hip, there is no difficulty in making this diagnosis radiographically if the chondroid bodies are ossified sufficiently to be recognized. However, if the bodies are not ossified, the clinical history must be used to suggest the diagnosis. The knee joint with its surrounding bursae and recesses is far more expansile than the hip joint. Therefore, the bones within the joint will not be affected except to develop secondary mechanical osteoarthritis. If the clinical history suggests the diagnosis and the chondroid bodies cannot be identified on the radiograph, arthrography should be performed.

Pigmented Villonodular Synovitis (PVNS)

The knee is the most common joint involved in pigmented villonodular synovitis. The joint space tends to be maintained until late in the disease. PVNS tends to involve one compartment of the knee rather than the entire knee. Cystic changes develop in both the tibia and the adjacent femur. There is little evidence of bone repair or osteophyte formation. The age and single joint involvement help to confirm the diagnosis.

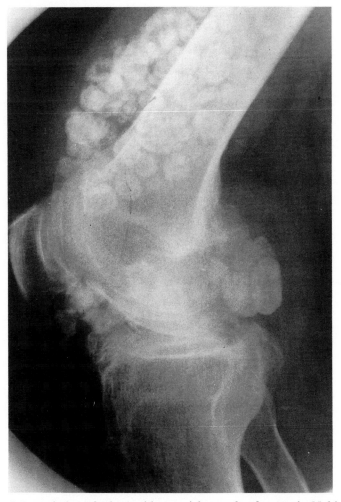

FIGURE 4–18. Lateral view of a knee with synovial osteochondromatosis. Multiple ossific bodies are seen throughout the knee joint.

SUGGESTED READINGS

Butt WP: Radiology of the infected joint. Clin Orthop Rel Res 96:136, 1973.

Gilbert M, Cockin J: An evaluation of the radiological changes in haemophilic arthropathy of the knee. *In* Ala F, Dense WE (eds): Proceedings of the 7th Congress of the World Federation of Haemophilia. Amsterdam, Excerpta Medica, 1973, p 191.

Goldman AB: Some miscellaneous joint diseases. Sem Roentgenol 17(1):60–80, 1982.

Lagier R: Femoral cortical erosions and osteoarthrosis of the knee in chondrocalcinosis. An anatomo-radiological study of two cases. Fortschr Geb Rontgenstr Nuklearmed 120:460–467, 1974.

Martel W, Holt JF, Cassidy JT: Roentgenologic manifestations of juvenile rheumatoid arthritis. AJR 88:400, 1962.

Milgram JW: Radiological and pathologic manifestations of osteochondritis dissecans of the distal femur. A study of 50 cases. Radiology 126:305, 1978.

Resnick D, Niwayama G: The "target area" approach to articular disorders: A synopsis. *In* Resnick D, Niwayama G (eds): Diagnosis of Bone and Joint Disorders, Vol 3. Philadelphia, W. B. Saunders Company, 1981.

Resnick D, Niwayama G, Goergen TG, et al.: Clinical, radiographic and pathologic abnormalities in calcium pyrophosphate dihydrate deposition disease (CPPD): Pseudogout. Radiology 122:1–15, 1977.

Scott PM: Bone lesions in pigmented villonodular synovitis. J Bone Joint Surg 50B:306, 1968.

Thomas R, Resnick D, Alazraki N, et al.: Compartmental evaluation in osteoarthritis of the knee: Comparison of diagnostic modalities. Radiology 116:585–594, 1975.

Williams JL, Cliff MM, Bonakdurpour A: Spontaneous osteonecrosis of the knee. Radiology 107:15, 1973.

Zimmerman C, Sayegh V: Roentgen manifestations of synovial osteochondromatosis. AJR 83:680, 1960.

chapter 5

APPROACH TO THE SHOULDER

Pain in the shoulder is a common problem affecting all ages of the general population. It is the second most common cause of musculoskeletal pain. Radiographic diagnosis of the disease entity causing non-specific pain begins with evaluation of how the shoulder joint has been affected. There are three areas in the shoulder joint to be observed: (1) the glenohumeral joint, (2) the subacromial space, and (3) the acromioclavicular joint.

GLENOHUMERAL JOINT INVOLVEMENT

Narrowing of the glenohumeral joint space with lack of involvement of the acromioclavicular (AC) joint or the subacromial space is usually accompanied by radiographic changes of osteoarthritis. It must be remembered that the shoulder is not a weight-bearing joint and therefore will not spontaneously develop primary or mechanical osteoarthritis. Osteoarthritic changes superimposed on glenohumeral joint space narrowing indicate a primary underlying abnormality in the cartilage. This abnormality may be disruption, deformity, or deposition.

Disruption of the cartilage can occur either in chronic repetitive trauma, such as recurrent dislocations, or in late-stage osteonecrosis. In the post-traumatic shoulder, a Hill-Sachs deformity, a "trough sign," and/or a Bankart lesion may be identified in addition to the glenohumeral joint space narrowing and osteoarthritic changes. In late-stage osteonecrosis the humeral head will be flattened and often fragmented.

Distortion of the underlying cartilage occurs in epiphyseal dysplasia or dysplasia of the scapular neck. In both instances the glenohumeral joint space narrowing and osteoarthritic changes will be superimposed on a recognizably dysplastic humeral head or flattened glenoid.

Deposition of a foreign substance into the cartilage is the most common cause of cartilage degeneration. This is observed in crystalline deposition disease, acromegaly, and ochronosis. The most common of these is calcium pyrophosphate dihydrate (CPPD) crystal deposition disease.

Calcium Pyrophosphate Dihydrate (CPPD) Crystal Deposition Disease (Fig. 5–1)

Observation of osteoarthritis involving both glenohumeral joints in a patient strongly suggests CPPD arthropathy. Early, before the joint is narrowed, chondrocalcinosis may be identified. With glenohumeral joint space narrowing, one will see subchondral sclerosis, osteophytosis, and occasionally cyst formation. The osteophyte will be seen best on the external rotation AP view. One may be able to identify calcification in the cartilage of the AC joint, making the diagnosis more definitive.

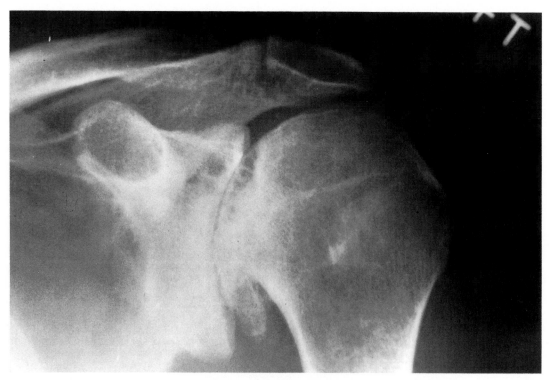

FIGURE 5–1. AP view of the shoulder in CPPD arthropathy. There is narrowing of the glenohumeral joint space with preservation of the subacromial and acromio-clavicular joint spaces. A huge medial osteophyte is identified on the humeral head. There is subchondral sclerosis of both the humeral head and the glenoid.

THE SUBACROMIAL SPACE

Isolated loss of the subacromial space occurs in (1) a chronic rotator cuff tear and (2) certain positions in the shoulder impingement syndrome. If there is less than 7 mm between the undersurface of the acromion and the top of the humeral head, this space is considered narrowed.

Chronic Rotator Cuff Tear (Fig. 5–2)

The glenohumeral joint space is preserved. The humeral head appears superior to its normal articulation with the glenoid and the space between the acromion and humeral head measures less than 7 mm. There is osseous erosion of the undersurface of the acromion with adjacent bone sclerosis. There may be sclerosis of the articulating humeral head as well. These radiographic changes are seen only in a chronic tear. There are no plain film findings in an acute rotator cuff tear; the radiographic diagnosis must be made through another modality, such as arthrography, ultrasonography, or magnetic resonance imaging.

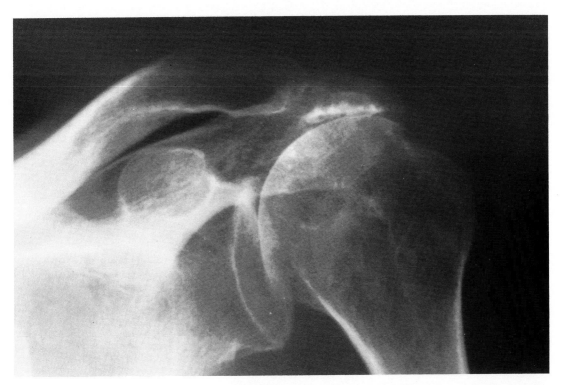

FIGURE 5–2. AP view of the shoulder demonstrating changes of a chronic rotator cuff tear. The glenohumeral joint space is preserved. The humeral head abuts the acromion. There is subchondral sclerosis of the undersurface of the acromion.

Shoulder Impingement Syndrome (Figs. 5–3 and 5–4)

In the shoulder impingement syndrome, pain is caused when the periarticular soft tissues such as the rotator cuff, biceps tendon, or subacromial bursa are trapped between the greater tuberosity of the humeral head and the coracoacromial ligamentous arch. Pain is produced on abduction or elevation of the externally rotated arm. On the normal AP view of the shoulder, bone excrescences are seen on the undersurface of the acromion (Fig. 5–3). These excrescences may be better visualized on an AP view in which the tube is angled 30 degrees caudally. Often there is some flattening, bone sclerosis, and bone proliferation at the greater tuberosity. If the shoulder is radiographed in external rotation and abduction, the greater tuberosity appears to abut the acromion (Fig. 5–4). Frequently, a coexistent chronic rotator cuff tear is present.

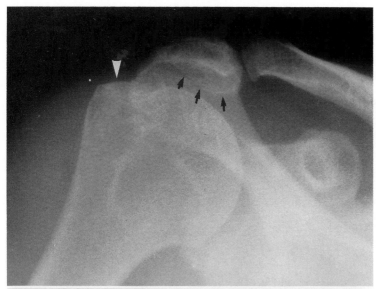

FIGURE 5–3. AP view of the shoulder in external rotation. The glenohumeral joint space is preserved. The subacromial joint space appears preserved. There is a bone excrescence seen on the undersurface of the acromion (arrows). There is adjacent sclerosis of the acromion. There is some flattening of the greater tuberosity where the rotator cuff attaches (arrowhead).

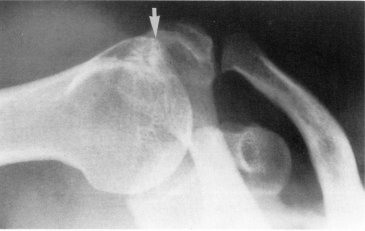

FIGURE 5–4. AP view of the same shoulder imaged in Figure 5–3 positioned in external rotation and abduction. The glenohumeral joint space is preserved. The greater tuberosity abuts the acromion. There are flattening and bone sclerosis of the greater tuberosity (arrow). The findings are consistent with the shoulder impingement syndrome.

THE ACROMIOCLAVICULAR JOINT

Trauma is the most frequent cause of radiographic changes in the acromioclavicular joint. Acute trauma may cause not only separation but also lysis of the distal end of the clavicle (Fig. 5–5). Osteoarthritis is the most common radiographic change seen at the acromioclavicular joint and is believed to be secondary to past or chronic trauma. CPPD arthropathy may involve the acromioclavicular joint with calcification of the cartilage and later osteoarthritic changes. Various systemic diseases, such as hyperparathyroidism and scleroderma, will cause resorption of the distal end of the clavicle.

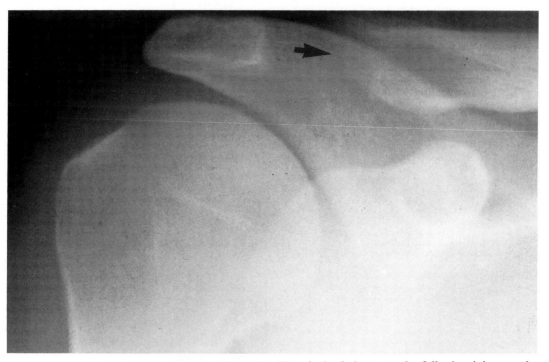

FIGURE 5–5. AP view of the shoulder obtained three months following injury to the acromioclavicular joint. The glenohumeral joint is preserved. The subacromial space is preserved. There is resorption of the distal end of the clavicle (arrow).

TOTAL COMPARTMENT INVOLVEMENT

Involvement of the glenohumeral, subacromial, and acromioclavicular joint spaces indicates an inflammatory arthropathy. However, the specific radiographic changes around these joint spaces distinguish one inflammatory arthropathy from another.

Rheumatoid Arthritis (Fig. 5–6)

When the shoulders are involved in rheumatoid arthritis, they are involved bilaterally and symmetrically. With loss of the glenohumeral joint space, the head moves inwardly; with involvement of the rotator cuff, the humeral head moves superiorly. Generalized osteoporosis is present. If erosions are present, they are usually juxta-articular on the humeral head. The distal end of the clavicle is tapered. There is no evidence of bone sclerosis or osteophyte formation.

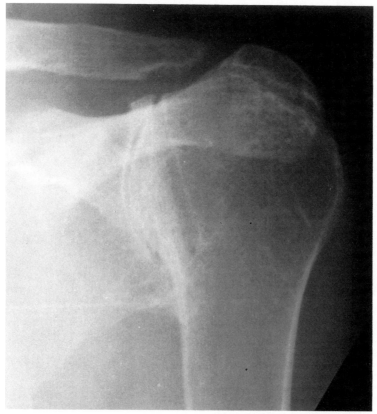

FIGURE 5–6. AP view of the shoulder in rheumatoid arthritis. There is generalized osteoporosis present. The humeral head has migrated inwardly and superiorly owing to loss of cartilage in the glenohumeral joint and the subacromial joint. There is erosion of the distal end of the clavicle.

Psoriatic Arthritis (Fig. 5–7)

In psoriatic arthritis, the shoulders are involved bilaterally but asymmetrically. The mineralization tends to be maintained. While there is cartilage loss, erosive disease is usually less prominent than bone proliferation. Ossification occurs at the rotator cuff attachment and the coracoclavicular ligament.

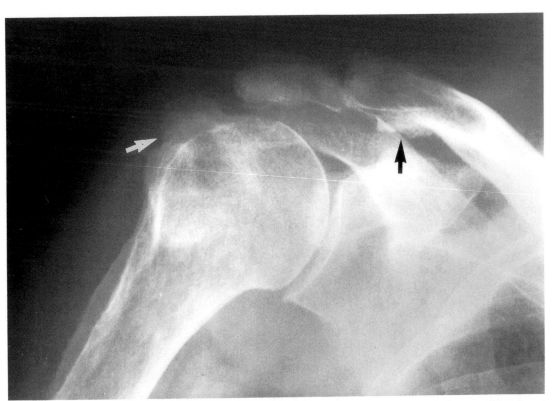

FIGURE 5–7. AP view of the shoulder in psoriatic arthritis. There is bone proliferation at the rotator cuff attachment and the coracoclavicular ligament (arrows). (From Brower AC: The radiographic features of psoriatic arthritis. *In* Gerber L, Espinoza L (eds): Psoriatic Arthritis. Orlando, FL, Grune & Stratton, Inc, 1985, p. 125.)

Ankylosing Spondylitis (Fig. 5–8)

The shoulder may be affected in two ways in ankylosing spondylitis. The most common finding is relatively early ankylosis without evidence of erosive disease. However, in some individuals there may be a large erosion of the superolateral aspect of the humeral head, described as a "hatchet" deformity. Ankylosis may be superimposed on this hatchet-like erosion.

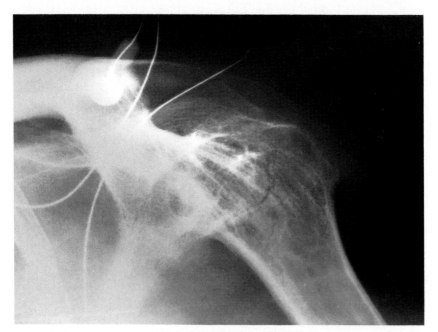

FIGURE 5–8. AP view of the shoulder in long-standing ankylosing spondylitis. The humeral head is ankylosed to the glenoid. There is extensive ossification of the coracoclavicular ligament.

Bleeding Abnormalities (Fig. 5–9)

While the inflammatory processes cause a loss of all of the potential joint spaces in the shoulder, blood within the joint will initially create a widening of all of the joint spaces visualized. This can be seen after acute trauma, in hemophilia, and in patients placed on anticoagulants. In these cases the humeral head lies inferiorly and laterally in relation to the glenoid. In hemophilia one may detect overgrowth of the humeral head and cystic changes on both sides of the joint secondary to intraosseous bleeding.

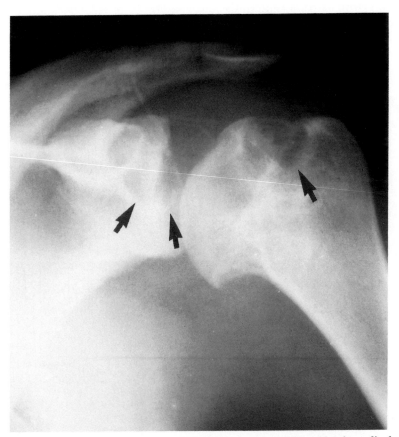

FIGURE 5–9. AP view of the shoulder in hemophilia. The humeral head has been displaced inferiorly and laterally from its normal articulation with the glenoid. This is secondary to hemarthrosis. There are cystic changes in the glenoid and the humeral head consistent with intraosseous bleeding (arrows).

NORMAL JOINT SPACE

Two painful disorders of the shoulders do not cause change in any joint space early on. These are hydroxyapatite deposition disease and osteonecrosis.

Hydroxyapatite Deposition Disease (HADD) (Figs. 5–10 and 5–11)

Hydroxyapatite deposition disease, commonly known as calcific tendinitis or bursitis, is the most common cause of shoulder pain. It is present in 40 per cent of painful shoulders. It appears as amorphous calcification in one of the tendons surrounding the shoulder joint. One can usually identify which tendon is involved by observing the change in position of the calcification between internal and external rotation views. The calcification may break out of the tendon and deposit in the bursa. Some patients with chronic tendinitis and bursitis have degeneration of the rotator cuff. In such cases, one may see the changes of a chronic rotator cuff tear. Degeneration of the glenohumeral joint space has also been described with secondary osteoarthritis in the late phases of this disease.

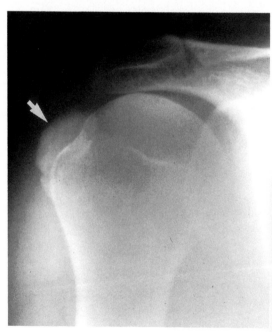

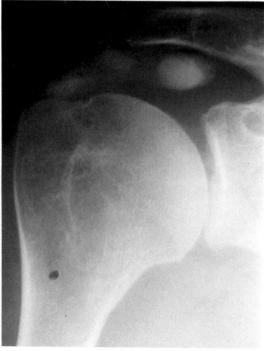

FIGURE 5–10. AP view of the shoulder showing normal glenohumeral, subacromial, and acromioclavicular joint spaces. There are no significant bone abnormalities. There is a large amorphous calcific deposit seen in the area of the rotator cuff attachment (arrow).

FIGURE 5–11. AP view of the shoulder demonstrating amorphous calcification in the rotator cuff attachment and subacromial bursa.

Osteonecrosis (Fig. 5–12)

Osteonecrosis of the shoulder, as of any other joint, is a disorder of the bone and not of the cartilage. Therefore, in the early phases no change occurs in the joint space. The first radiographic manifestation of osteonecrosis is smudging of the trabecular pattern near the articular surface of the humeral head. This is usually followed by a subchondral lucency beneath the articular surface, indicating imminent collapse of the articular bone into the bone beneath. Once collapse has occurred there is disruption of the cartilage over the humeral head and the appearance of secondary osteoarthritic changes.

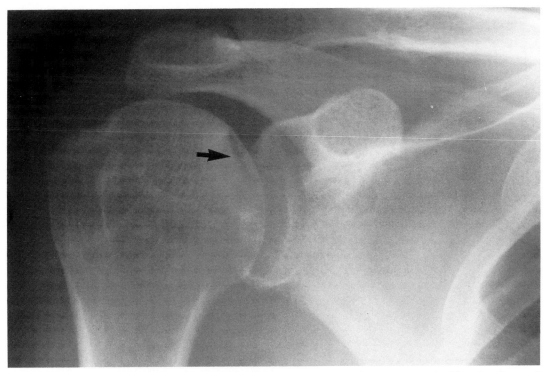

FIGURE 5–12. AP view of the shoulder demonstrating osteonecrosis. The glenohumeral, subacromial, and acromioclavicular joint spaces are maintained. There is subchondral bone sclerosis of the humeral head. There is a subchondral lucency present, indicating a subchondral fracture (arrow).

SUGGESTED READINGS

Bonavita J, Dalinka MK, Schumacher HR Jr: Hydroxyapatite deposition disease. Radiology 134:621–625, 1980.

Cone RO, Resnick D: Degenerative disease of the shoulder. Australas Radiol 28:232–239, 1984.

Cone RO, Resnick D, Danzig L: Shoulder impingement syndrome: Radiographic evaluation. Radiology 150:29–33, 1984.

Kerr R, Resnick D, Pineda C, Haghighi P: Osteoarthritis of the glenohumeral joint: A radiologic-pathologic study. AJR 144:967–972, 1985.

Kotzen LM: Roentgen diagnosis of rotator cuff tear. Report of 48 surgically proven cases. AJR 112:507, 1971.

McCarty DJ, Halverson PB, Carrera GF, et al.: "Milwaukee shoulder"—association of microspheroids containing hydroxyapatite crystals, active collagenase and neutral protease with rotator cuff defects. 1. Clinical aspects. Arthritis Rheum 24:464–473, 1981.

Peterson CC Jr, Silbiger ML: Reiter's syndrome and psoriatic arthritis: Their roentgen spectra and some interesting similarities. AJR 101:860, 1967.

Petersson CJ, Redlund-Johnell I: Joint space in normal glenohumeral radiographs. Acta Orthop Scand 54:274–276, 1983.

Resnick D: Patterns of peripheral joint disease in ankylosing spondylitis. Radiology 110:523, 1974.

Sbarbaro JL: The rheumatoid shoulder. Orthop Clin North Am 6:593, 1975.

chapter 6

THE
SACROILIAC
JOINT

The sacroiliac (SI) joint is perhaps the most difficult joint in the skeleton to image adequately to make an accurate diagnosis of a disorder affecting it. This is partially due to (1) obscuration of the joint by multiple overlying soft tissue structures and (2) variations in the obliquity of the joint within an individual and among individuals. A modified AP Ferguson view (see Chapter 1) is the most useful view to eliminate the confusing soft tissue shadows and to profile that part of the joint which is affected by all disease processes.

The SI joint consists of two parts: (1) the true joint and (2) the ligamentous attachment between the two adjacent bones (Fig. 6–1). The anterior, inferior one half to two thirds of the SI joint is a true synovial joint. The iliac side is covered by hyaline cartilage 1 mm in thickness; the sacral side is covered by fibrous cartilage that varies from 3 to 5 mm in thickness. Owing to the thinness of the cartilage on the iliac side compared to the sacral side, all disease processes involve the iliac side first and the sacral side second. The cartilage-covered area is surrounded by synovium. The posterior, superior portion of the SI joint is nothing more than a cleft between the sacrum and the ilium. There is no cartilage covering either bone in this area. Intraosseous ligaments extend between the sacrum and ilium, joining the two bones together. The AP modified Ferguson view images the anterior, inferior–most aspect of the SI joint, the area where disease first begins.

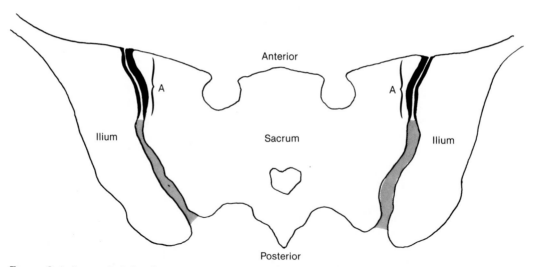

FIGURE 6–1. Anatomical drawing of the sacroiliac joints as viewed in an axial plane. The true synovial joint (A) is seen as the anterior one third of the cleft between the two bones. Note that the cartilage on the iliac side is thinner than the cartilage on the sacral side. The posterior portion of the cleft has no cartilage or synovium. Intraosseous ligaments join the sacrum to the ilium.

The obliquity of the SI joint varies from person to person. Therefore, no two individuals have identical-appearing SI joints. There are two criteria for determining normality of an SI joint. First, although the width of the SI joint varies from person to person according to the thickness of the cartilage on the sacral side, the SI joint should be of uniform width within the individual. Second, the white cortical line along the iliac and sacral side should be intact (Fig. 6–2). If these criteria are not met, the SI joint must be considered abnormal. The diagnosis of disease involving the sacroiliac joint depends upon observing the following: (1) the width of the joint space, (2) the presence and type of erosions, (3) the presence and type of sclerosis, (4) the presence and type of bone bridging, and (5) the distribution of the above changes.

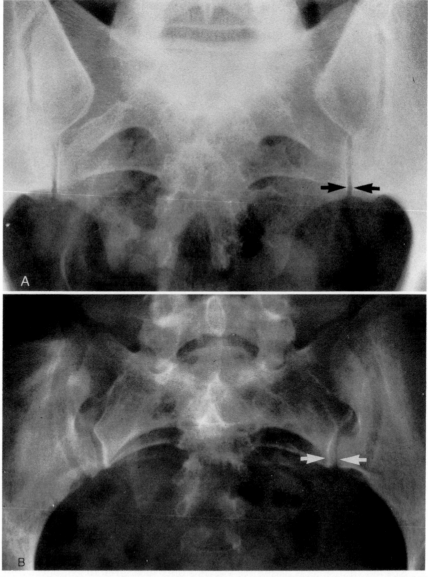

FIGURE 6–2. *A,* Normal AP view of the SI joints in a male. *B,* Normal AP view of the SI joints in a female. Note that in both cases the joint is of uniform width and the white cortical line (arrows) along the joint margins is intact. (*B* From Brower AC: Disorders of the sacroiliac joint. Radiolog 1(20):3, 1978.)

WIDTH OF THE JOINT SPACE

Apparent widening of the SI joint is observed with infection and the inflammatory spondyloarthropathies. Uniform narrowing of the SI joint is observed in rheumatoid arthritis. Irregularity of the width of the SI joint, where parts are too narrow and other parts are too wide, is observed in the crystalline arthropathies and in osteoarthritis.

PRESENCE AND TYPES OF EROSIONS

Erosions are present in all of the inflammatory arthropathies. Small and succinct erosions tend to be present in ankylosing spondylitis and rheumatoid arthritis, whereas large and extensive erosions tend to be present in psoriatic, Reiter's, and septic arthritis. A large erosion may occur in gout, but it will have a sclerotic well-defined border as opposed to the ill-defined border seen in the inflammatory arthropathies. Erosions are not seen in CPPD or osteoarthritis.

PRESENCE AND TYPE OF SCLEROSIS

Reparative bone is seen behind or adjacent to erosive changes. This sclerosis tends to be minimal in ankylosing spondylitis and much more extensive in Reiter's, psoriatic, and septic arthritis. Reparative bone is seen in CPPD, gout, and osteoarthritis. This sclerosis abuts the articular surface, usually at the inferior and superior aspects of the true joint. Sclerosis is seen in a wedge-shaped configuration on the iliac side of the SI joint in osteitis condensans ilii. The widest part of the wedge is along the inferior aspect of the ilium.

PRESENCE AND TYPE OF BONE BRIDGING

There are two types of bone bridging: (a) true bone ankylosis of the joint itself and (b) anterior osteophyte formation bridging across the ilium to the sacrum anterior to the joint. Bone ankylosis is seen in the inflammatory arthropathies and in septic arthritis. Anterior osteophyte formation is seen in the crystalline arthropathies and osteoarthritis.

DISTRIBUTION OF CHANGES

Disease entities are either unilateral, bilateral and symmetrical, or bilateral and asymmetrical. Septic arthritis is almost always unilateral. Ankylosing spondylitis, spondylitis associated with bowel disease, CPPD, and osteitis condensans ilii tend to be bilateral and symmetrical. Psoriatic arthritis, Reiter's disease, gout, and osteoarthritis tend to be bilateral and asymmetrical.

The most significant disorders of the SI joint are the inflammatory ones. Therefore, knowledge of radiographic changes occurring in these disorders is important. All of the inflammatory disease processes affect the SI joint in a specific sequence varying only in degree of change within the sequence. Erosive changes begin on the iliac side of the SI joint. The earliest change observed is poor definition or loss of the white cortical line on the iliac side (Fig. 6–3). As the erosive disease progresses, the SI joint becomes apparently widened (Fig. 6–4). The body then responds by laying down reparative bone behind the erosive changes (Fig. 6–5). The reparative process then becomes the dominant part of the radiographic picture. Following this, bone ankylosis occurs across the SI joint (Fig. 6–6). Once the SI joint is ankylosed, the surrounding bone becomes osteoporotic secondary to loss of normal mechanical stress across the SI joint (Fig. 6–7). Although each inflammatory disease process goes through this sequence of events, disease entities can be distinguished through their extent and distribution of involvement. Specific disorders of the SI joints and their distinguishing radiographic characteristics are now illustrated and discussed.

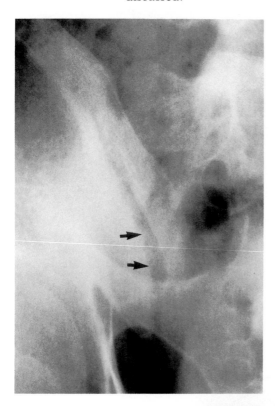

FIGURE 6–3. AP Ferguson view of the SI joint. The white cortical line is intact on the sacral side. It is ill defined on the iliac side (arrows).

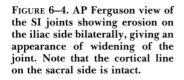

FIGURE 6–4. AP Ferguson view of the SI joints showing erosion on the iliac side bilaterally, giving an appearance of widening of the joint. Note that the cortical line on the sacral side is intact.

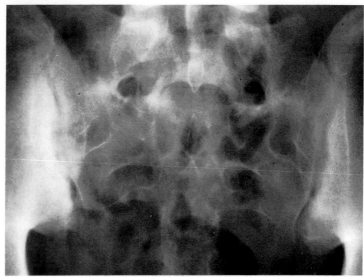

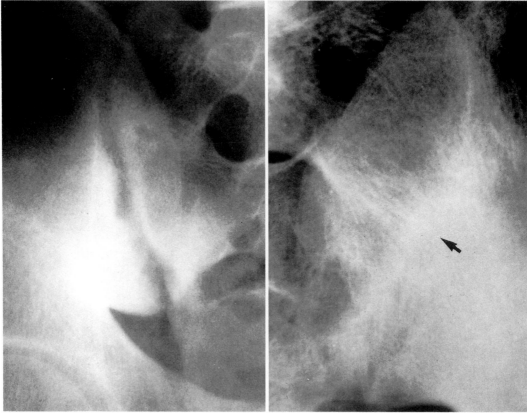

FIGURE 6–5   FIGURE 6–6

FIGURE 6–5. AP Ferguson view of an SI joint showing extensive erosive changes on both the iliac and sacral sides. There is extensive bone repair behind the erosive changes on both sides.

FIGURE 6–6. AP Ferguson view of the SI joint showing bone ankylosis (arrow) across the sacroiliac joint.

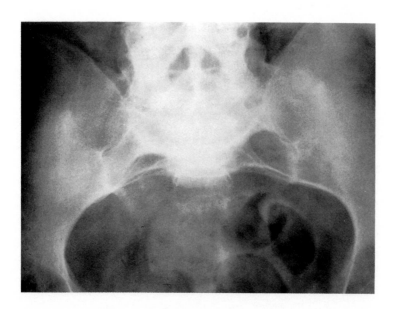

FIGURE 6–7. AP view of the sacroiliac joints showing total bone ankylosis across the joints and secondary osteoporosis.

Ankylosing Spondylitis (Figs. 6–8 and 6–9)

The first radiographic change observed in ankylosing spondylitis is found in the SI joints. It involves the joints bilaterally and symmetrically. The erosions appear to be small and succinct, presenting an edge that has been likened to the perforated edge of a postage stamp (Fig. 6–8). The amount of sclerosis, or bone repair, is also somewhat limited. Rather early in the disease, before the erosions or sclerosis becomes too extensive, bone ankylosis takes place. The ankylosis occurs not only in the true synovial aspect of the joint but also in the posterior superior cleft of the joint (Fig. 6–9). Ankylosing spondylitis is an ossifying disease; it will ossify the ligaments that join the sacrum to the ilium in the posterior superior aspect of the joint. Radiographically this is seen as a star with radiations from its center. A similar sequence of changes is observed in the arthropathy associated with bowel disease.

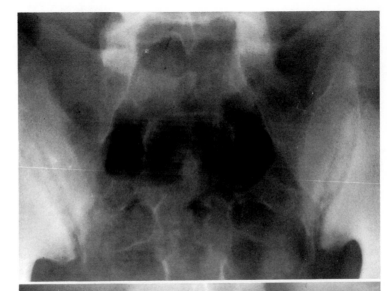

FIGURE 6–8. AP Ferguson view of the SI joints in a patient with ankylosing spondylitis. There is bilateral symmetrical involvement. There are small succinct erosions involving both sides of the joint with limited bone repair. (From Brower AC: Disorders of the sacroiliac joint. Radiolog 1(20):3, 1978.)

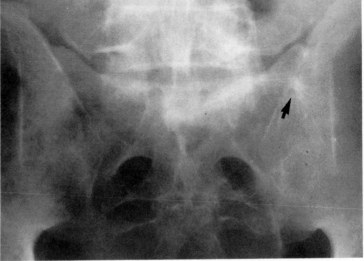

FIGURE 6–9. An AP view of the sacroiliac joints in long-standing ankylosing spondylitis. Both sacroiliac joints are completely ankylosed. A "start" is seen at the superior aspect of the joint (arrow) representing ossification of the ligaments between the sacrum and the ilium. (From Brower AC: Disorders of the sacroiliac joint. Radiolog 1(20):3, 1978.)

Psoriatic Arthritis and Reiter's Disease
(Figs. 6–10 and 6–11)

One cannot distinguish psoriatic arthritis from Reiter's disease in observing the radiographic changes in the SI joint. Both present involvement of the SI joints in a bilateral and asymmetrical fashion (Fig. 6–10). The erosive component appears to be much more extensive than that seen in ankylosing spondylitis (Fig. 6–11). Likewise, the bone repair is more extensive. Ankylosis may or may not occur, but when it does, it occurs later in the disease process. Because the disease process is usually bilateral and asymmetrical, in the early stages it may present as unilateral involvement, which may be subtle. Scintigraphy may be useful in distinguishing true unilateral disease from subtle bilateral, asymmetrical disease. However, once the changes become obvious on one side there should be subtle changes involving the opposite side as well.

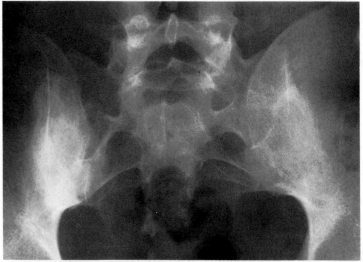

FIGURE 6–10. An AP view of the sacroiliac joints in a patient with psoriatic arthritis. There is bilateral asymmetrical involvement. There is ankylosis of the left sacroiliac joint. The right sacroiliac joint shows erosive changes with extensive bone repair. Ankylosis is beginning to occur.

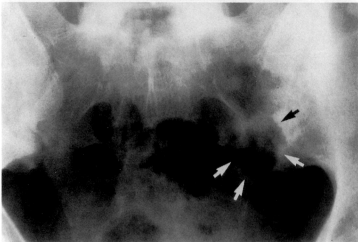

FIGURE 6–11. An AP view of the sacroiliac joints in a patient with Reiter's disease. There is bilateral asymmetrical involvement. The right sacroiliac joint shows small erosive changes with reparative bone formation. The left sacroiliac joint shows a large erosion (arrows) with patchier bone repair. (From Brower AC: Disorders of the sacroiliac joint. Radiolog 1(20):3, 1978.)

Rheumatoid Arthritis (Figs. 6–12 to 6–14)

Rheumatoid arthritis causes symmetrical uniform narrowing of the SI joint with very little reparative bone and no evidence of osteophyte formation (Fig. 6–12). Occasionally erosive disease may be present but never to the extent of presenting a widened joint space as seen in the spondyloarthropathies (Fig. 6–13). Bone ankylosis may occur, but this will be present in the synovial aspect of the joint only (Fig. 6–14). In contrast to the spondyloarthropathies, there is no ossification of the ligaments connecting the sacrum to the ilium. Involvement of the SI joints occurs late in rheumatoid arthritis and frequently goes unobserved because of the extensive involvement of the appendicular joints.

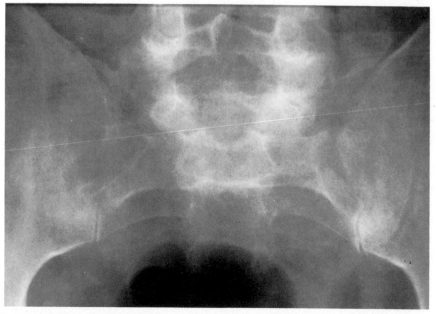

FIGURE 6–12. An AP view of the sacroiliac joints in a patient with rheumatoid arthritis. There is bilateral symmetrical involvement with narrowing of both sacroiliac joints. No erosions are seen. There is minimal sclerosis around the left SI joint.

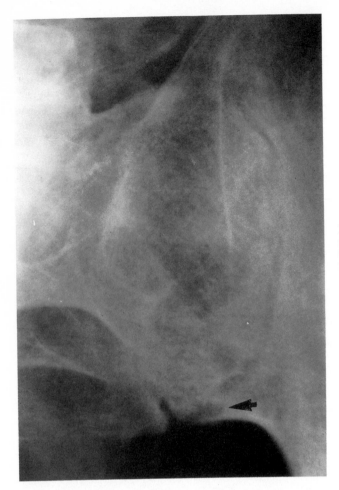

FIGURE 6–13. An AP view of a sacroiliac joint in a patient with rheumatoid arthritis. Inferiorly there is a small erosion (arrow) without reparative response.

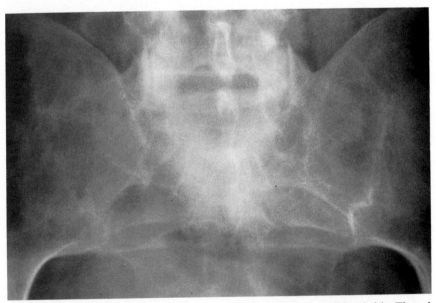

FIGURE 6–14. An AP view of the SI joints in a patient with rheumatoid arthritis. There is bilateral bone ankylosis of the synovial part of the sacroiliac joint. There is no evidence of ligamentous ossification.

Infection (Figs. 6–15 to 6–17)

Septic arthritis is almost always unilateral in distribution. It leads to extensive erosion and extensive bone repair and may involve more than just the synovial aspect of the joint (Fig. 6–15). Tuberculous septic arthritis may cause the formation of a calcified abscess anterior to the SI joint (Fig. 6–16). Bone ankylosis may result from septic arthritis; septic arthritis is the most common cause of unilateral sacroiliac ankylosis (Fig. 6–17).

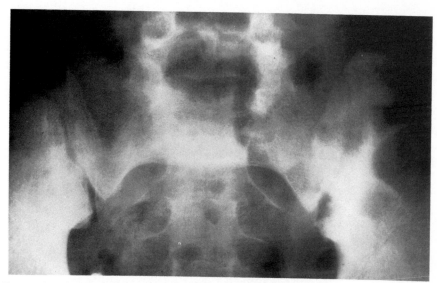

FIGURE 6–15. An AP view of the sacroiliac joints in a patient with septic arthritis. The right sacroiliac joint is entirely normal. The left sacroiliac joint shows erosive changes inferiorly and extensive bone repair surrounding the erosive changes. (From Brower AC: Disorders of the sacroiliac joint. Radiolog 1(20):3, 1978.)

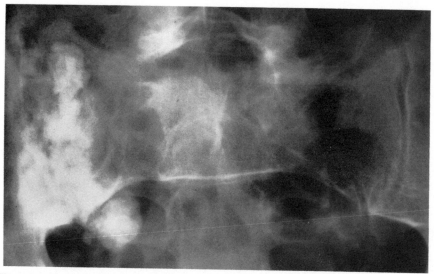

FIGURE 6–16. An AP view of the sacroiliac joints in a patient with tuberculous septic arthritis. The left sacroiliac joint is normal. The right SI joint is obscured by a calcified abscess anterior to the sacroiliac joint.

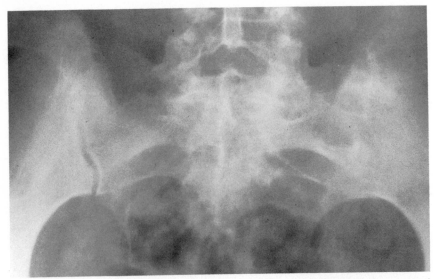

FIGURE 6–17. An AP view of the sacroiliac joints in a patient with previously known septic arthritis. The right sacroiliac joint is normal. The left sacroiliac joint is completely ankylosed. (From Brower AC: Disorders of the sacroiliac joint. Radiolog 1(20):3, 1978.)

Gout (Fig. 6–18)

Deposit of urate crystals into the cartilage leads to irregular loss of the joint space and superimposed osteoarthritic changes. In this instance it is impossible to distinguish gout from osteoarthritis. A tophus may form at the SI joint and create a large erosion of the anterior inferior aspect of the SI joint. However, this erosion, like those associated with tophi elsewhere, has a well-defined sclerotic border and occasionally an overhanging edge of cortex. Seven per cent of the patients with radiographic gout demonstrate this classic lesion.

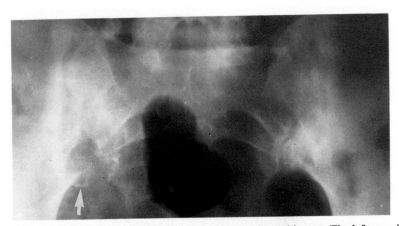

FIGURE 6–18. An AP view of the sacroiliac joints in a patient with gout. The left sacroiliac joint shows changes of degenerative arthritis. There is patchy sclerosis on the iliac side. There is irregularity to the width of the joint space. The white cortical line on the sacral side is maintained. The right sacroiliac joint has a large erosion inferiorly. The erosion has a sclerotic rim and an overhanging edge of cortex (arrow). The erosion is classical of that produced by a tophus. (From Brower AC: Disorders of the sacroiliac joint. Radiolog 1(20):3, 1978.)

Calcium Pyrophosphate Dihydrate (CPPD) Crystal Deposition Disease (Fig. 6–19)

The diagnosis of CPPD can be made when one sees calcification of the articular cartilage in both SI joints. This tends to be symmetrical when present. Should arthropathy develop secondary to this deposition, one may see air, or a vacuum phenomenon, within the SI joint. Eventually osteoarthritic changes may be seen (see Osteoarthritis).

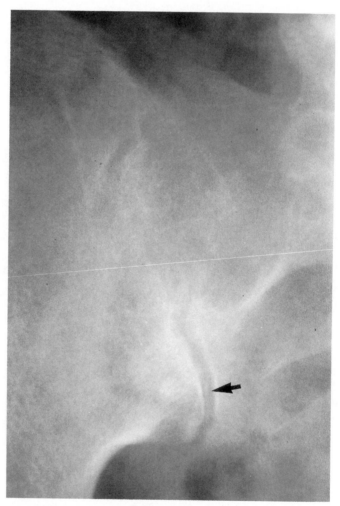

FIGURE 6–19. An AP view of the sacroiliac joint in a patient with CPPD. Calcification (arrow) is seen within the inferior aspect of the joint.

Osteoarthritis (Figs. 6–20 to 6–22)

Osteoarthritis of the SI joints is a degeneration of the cartilage and associated bone changes secondary to abnormal mechanical stress across the joint. It is most commonly seen in males, especially those involved in heavy labor. It may be bilateral and asymmetrical, or unilateral. Irregular narrowing of the sacroiliac joint is observed to be most pronounced at the superior and inferior aspects of the true synovial joint (Fig. 6–20). Along with the narrowing, subchondral sclerosis develops in these areas. Erosive changes are not part of this arthropathy. Large osteophytes may develop superiorly and inferiorly and bridge the ilium to the sacrum anterior to the actual joint. One may confuse this osteophyte formation with true bone ankylosis (Fig. 6–21). However, observation of part of the joint as normal should eliminate this confusing possibility. If necessary, a CT scan can be performed and demonstrate its anterior location (Fig. 6–22).

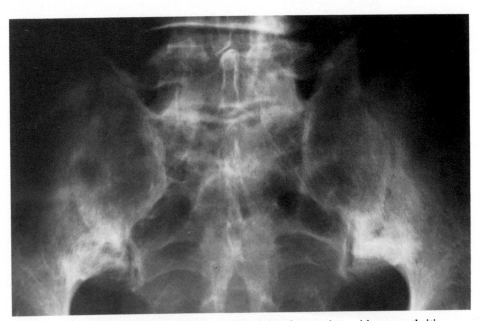

FIGURE 6–20. AP Ferguson view of the sacroiliac joints in a patient with osteoarthritis. There is bilateral asymmetrical involvement. The right sacroiliac joint shows sclerosis in the inferior aspect of the joint. The joint margin is still defined. There is bone bridging inferiorly by a large anterior osteophyte. The left sacroiliac joint is irregularly narrowed. There is sclerosis present inferiorly and superiorly in the joint. There is irregular bone bridging. (From Brower AC: Disorders of the sacroiliac joint. Radiolog 1(20):3, 1978.)

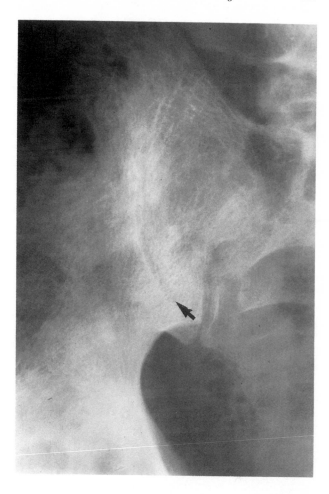

FIGURE 6–21. An AP view of a sacroiliac joint in a patient with osteoarthritis. The inferior aspect of the joint is well maintained. There is sclerosis on the iliac side on the inferior and superior aspects of the joint. There is bridging by an anterior osteophyte extending from the ilium to the sacrum (arrow). This might be confused with bone ankylosis.

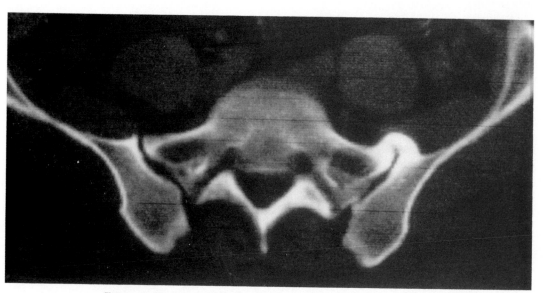

FIGURE 6–22. The sacroiliac joints in a patient with osteoarthritis as viewed by means of computed axial tomography. The right SI joint is within normal limits. The left SI joint shows bone sclerosis anteriorly and a large osteophyte bridging the space between the ilium and the sacrum anterior to the true joint.

Osteitis Condensans Ilii (Figs. 6–23 and 6–24)

This is a disorder that surrounds the SI joint but does not affect the joint itelf. It most commonly presents in multiparous females as a dome-shaped area of sclerosis on the iliac side of the SI joint. The widest portion of the sclerosis is found in the inferior aspect of the ilium (Fig. 6–23). There may be some sclerosis on the sacral side but always to a lesser extent than on the iliac side. It can be seen in males as well. It is believed to result from stress to this area secondary to instability at the pubic symphysis. Pain is usually present when the pubic symphysis is unstable. This instability can be demonstrated by "flamingo" views in which shifting weight from one leg to another shifts the apposition of the pubic rami (Fig. 6–24). Once the pubic symphysis is stabilized, either through surgery or through cessation of the activity that caused the instability, pain is no longer present. However, the radiographic changes may still be present. With time and continued pubic symphysis stability, the osteitis condensans ilii eventually resolves, with the iliac bone returning to normal.

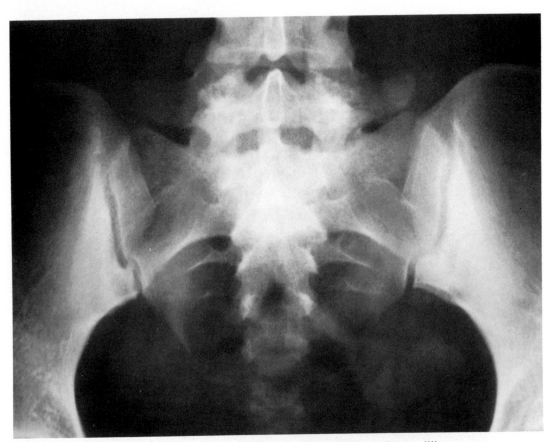

FIGURE 6–23. An AP view of the sacroiliac joints in a patient with osteitis condensans ilii. There is bilateral symmetrical involvement. The actual joint spaces are normal. There is a triangular homogeneous sclerosis involving the iliac side of the joint. (From Brower AC: Disorders of the sacroiliac joint. Radiolog 1(20):3, 1978.)

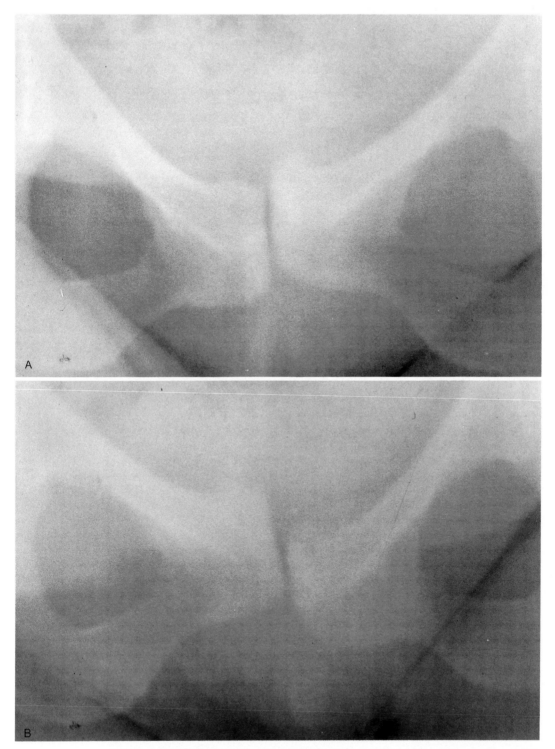

FIGURE 6–24. Instability of the pubic symphysis in a patient with osteitis condensans ilii. The instability is demonstrated by shifting weight from one leg to the other (A to B), causing a shift in the position of the pubic rami.

SUGGESTED READINGS

Berens DL: Roentgen features of ankylosing spondylitis. Clin Orthop 74:20–33, 1971.

Brower A: Disorders of the sacroiliac joint. Radiolog 1(20):3–26, 1978.

Dixon A St J, Lience E: Sacroiliac joint in adult rheumatoid arthritis and psoriatic arthropathy. Ann Rheum Dis 20:247–256, 1961.

Gillespie HW, Lloyd-Roberts G: Osteitis condensans. Br J Radiol 26:16–21, 1953.

Harris NH, Murray RO: Lesions of the symphysis in athletes. Br Med J 4:211, 1974.

Jajic I: Radiological changes in the sacroiliac joints and spine of patients with psoriatic arthritis and psoriasis. Ann Rheum Dis 27:1–6, 1968.

Malawista SE, Seegmiller JE, Hathaway BE, et al.: Sacroiliac gout. JAMA 194:954–956, 1965.

Numaguchi Y: Osteitis condensans ilii, including its resolution. Radiology 98:1–8, 1971.

Resnick D: Disorders of the axial skeleton which are lesser known, poorly recognized or misunderstood. Bull Rheum Dis 28:932–939, 1977-78.

Resnick D, Niwayama G, Georgen TG: Degenerative disease of the sacroiliac joint. Invest Radiol 10:608–621, 1975.

Resnick D, Niwayama G, Georgen TG: Comparison of radiographic abnormalities of the sacroiliac joint in degenerative disease and ankylosing spondylitis. AJR 128:189–196, 1977.

chapter 7

THE "PHYTES" OF THE SPINE

In evaluating the spine, one observes the size, shape, and mineralization of the different vertebral bodies. These parameters become abnormal in various systemic diseases. For example, a large vertebral body is seen in Paget's disease, a flattened vertebral body in eosinophilic granuloma, an H-shaped vertebral body in sickle cell disease, a sclerotic vertebral body in lymphoma, and an osteoporotic body in hyperparathyroidism. The arthropathies tend not to involve the vertebral body itself but primarily the apophyseal joints and the disc spaces. The most common arthropathy involving the apophyseal joints is osteoarthritis, which produces narrowing of the apophyseal joints, reparative bone, and osteophyte formation (Fig. 7–1). The inflammatory arthropathies cause erosive changes of the apophyseal joints, with or without eventual ankylosis. The inflammatory arthropathies may affect the disc space, but the most common disc space disorder is degeneration either idiopathically or secondary to abnormal deposition of material into the disc substance. Radiographic signs of disc degeneration are vacuum phenomenon, calcification, disc space narrowing, and reparative response in adjacent vertebral bodies.

However, many of the arthropathies lead to the development of various kinds of "phytes." The diagnosis of an arthropathy can be made through careful observation of the type of "phyte" that is produced. There are four different types of "phytes": (1) the syndesmophyte, (2) the marginal osteophyte, (3) the non-marginal osteophyte, and (4) the paraspinal phyte.

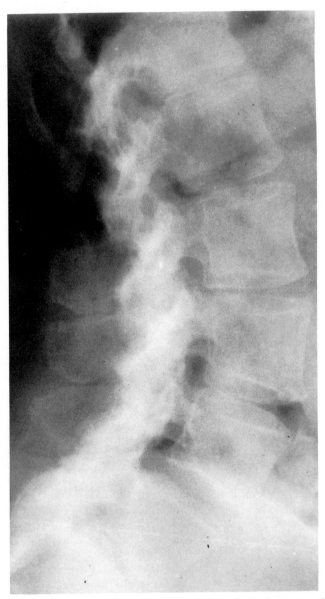

FIGURE 7–1. Lateral view of the lumbosacral spine in a patient with osteoarthritis of the apophyseal joints. Note the absence of osteophyte formation and bone sclerosis of the vertebral bodies. There is loss of the apophyseal joint spaces with extensive surrounding bone repair. (From Brower AC: The significance of various phytes of the spine. Radiolog 1(15):3, 1978.)

In order to understand the various kinds of "phytes" that distort the vertebral body and surround the disc, the anatomy of the disc interspace and surrounding soft tissues must be understood (Fig. 7–2). The central portion of the disc is known as the nucleus pulposus. This is surrounded by a fibrous ring called the anulus fibrosus. The nucleus pulposus and the inner portion of the anulus fibrosus are surrounded superiorly and inferiorly by the cartilaginous end-plate of the vertebral body. This cartilaginous vertebral end-plate does not extend to the borders of the bony vertebral body. Where the cartilaginous end-plate ends, the outermost fibers of the anulus fibrosus, called Sharpey's fibers, penetrate and connect the bone of one vertebral body to the bone of the adjacent vertebral body. The anterior longitudinal ligament adheres closely to the anterior border of the mid-portion of the vertebral body. At a level approximately 3 mm from the ends of the vertebral body, the anterior longitudinal ligament pulls away from the vertebral body and no longer closely adheres. It traverses the disc area in apposition to Sharpey's fibers and becomes closely adherent to the adjacent vertebral body 3 mm beyond the end-plate. The posterior longitudinal ligament adheres to the vertebral body in its entire length and is more intimately apposed to Sharpey's fibers posteriorly.

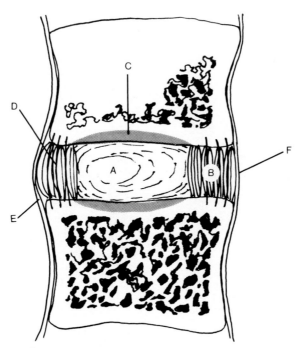

FIGURE 7–2. Anatomical drawing of the disc space and surrounding vertebral bodies. A = Nucleus pulposus; B = anulus fibrosus; C = cartilaginous portion of the vertebral end-plate; D = Sharpey's fibers; E = anterior longitudinal ligament; F = posterior longitudinal ligament.

SYNDESMOPHYTE

The syndesmophyte is a vertical ossification bridging two adjacent vertebral bodies (Fig. 7–3). It is the ossification of Sharpey's fibers of the anulus fibrosus. Since these fibers extend into the bone portion of the vertebral body, the syndesmophyte becomes a contiguous part of the vertebral bodies involved. The deep layers of the longitudinal ligaments may become ossified as well in forming this bridge. The syndesmophyte is the hallmark of ankylosing spondylitis. However, it may be seen in any of the spondyloarthropathies: Reiter's disease, psoriasis, and that associated with bowel disease.

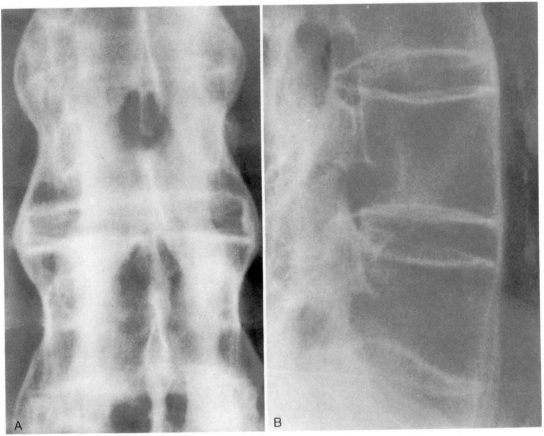

FIGURE 7–3. AP (A) and lateral (B) views of lumbar vertebral bodies jointed by syndesmophytes. At the disc level, the ossification is occurring in the anulus fibrosus and the deep layers of the anterior longitudinal ligament. (B from Brower AC: The significance of various phytes of the spine. Radiolog 1(15):3, 1978.)

MARGINAL OSTEOPHYTE

The marginal osteophyte is a horizontal bone extension of the vertebral end-plate (Fig. 7–4). It is an integral part of the vertebral body in that it has a medullary canal contiguous with the medullary canal of the vertebral body and cortex contiguous with the cortex of the vertebral body end-plate. Small marginal osteophytes are most commonly associated with degenerative disc disease and spondylosis deformans. Larger marginal osteophytes may turn from their horizontal course in a vertical direction and join with another marginal osteophyte from an adjacent vertebral body to form a bridge. These larger bridging marginal osteophytes are often post-traumatic but may be seen in combination with other types of "phytes" that are more diagnostic of the underlying disease entity.

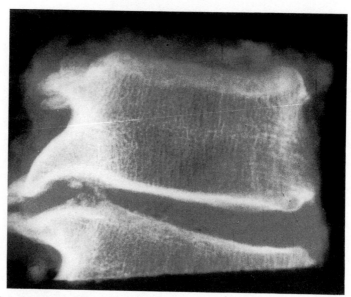

FIGURE 7–4. Specimen radiograph of disc space and surrounding vertebral bodies showing presence of marginal osteophytes. Note that the medullary portion of the osteophyte is contiguous with the medullary portion of the vertebral body and that the cortex of the osteophyte is contiguous with the cortex of the vertebral body.

NON-MARGINAL OSTEOPHYTE

A non-marginal osteophyte is a horizontal extension or osteophyte of the vertebral body observed 2 to 3 mm away from the actual vertebral end-plate (Fig. 7–5). Again, a non-marginal osteophyte appears to be an integral part of the vertebral body, with its medullary canal and cortex connecting with that of the vertebral body. Small ones are associated with degenerative disc disease and spondylosis deformans. These are called traction osteophytes and are believed to indicate an element of instability in the spine. Like the marginal osteophyte, the non-marginal osteophyte may also turn vertically and join a similar non-marginal osteophyte from an adjacent vertebral body (Fig. 7–6). These larger non-marginal osteophytes (sometimes called non-marginal syndesmophytes) are seen in psoriatic arthritis and Reiter's disease.

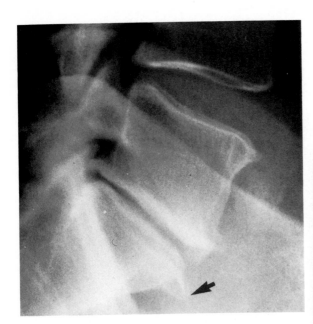

FIGURE 7–5. Lateral view of L5-S1 demonstrating a non-marginal osteophyte (arrow) on S1.

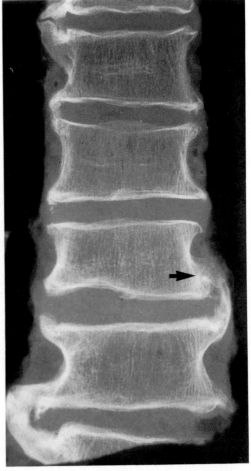

FIGURE 7–6. Specimen radiograph of disc and adjacent vertebral bodies demonstrating a large non-marginal osteophyte (arrow) joining a large marginal osteophyte.

PARASPINAL PHYTE

The paraspinal phyte is the ossification of the soft tissue structures that surround the vertebral body. This ossification is not an integral part of the vertebral body and can be separated from it (Fig. 7–7). Radiographically the paraspinal phyte is observed most often as ossification of a longitudinal ligament. A lucent line can be seen to separate this ossification from the cortex of the vertebral body. The paraspinal phyte is most commonly associated with diffuse idiopathic skeletal hyperostosis (DISH).

Having described the various "phytes" that occur around the spine, we will now discuss common specific disease entities that produce "phytes" and the type and location of the "phytes" produced.

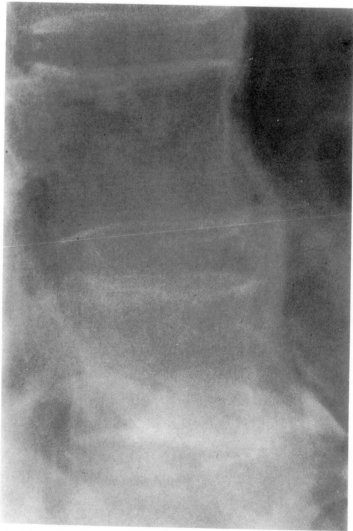

FIGURE 7–7. A lateral view of the lumbar spine demonstrating paraspinal phytes. This is ossification of the soft tissues and structures that surround the vertebral body. Note that these phytes are not a contiguous part of the vertebral body.

Degenerative Disc Disease—Primary and Secondary (Figs. 7–8 to 7–11)

Degenerative disc disease, or intervertebral osteochondrosis, is perhaps the most common positive radiogaphic finding in patients with back pain. If it occurs at one level, it is usually secondary to either the normal aging process or a premature aging process secondary to trauma. There is loss of normal resiliency of the nucleus pulposus and, with this, loss of normal disc height. As one observes the normal spine, the intervertebral disc spaces should increase as one descends the spine except at the level of C7-T1 and L5-S1, which are considered transitional areas. A disc space is considered narrow if the height is less than or equal to the one above it. Disc space narrowing is the most common radiographic sign of disc disease. Calcification and/or a vacuum phenomenon (air density) observed in a disc space is an absolute sign of disc degeneration. The vertebral bodies adjacent to the degenerated disc develop small marginal osteophytes and/or small non-marginal osteophytes along with a degree of subchondral bone repair (Fig. 7–8). The non-marginal osteophyte is called a traction osteophyte and indicates instability of the spine in this area.

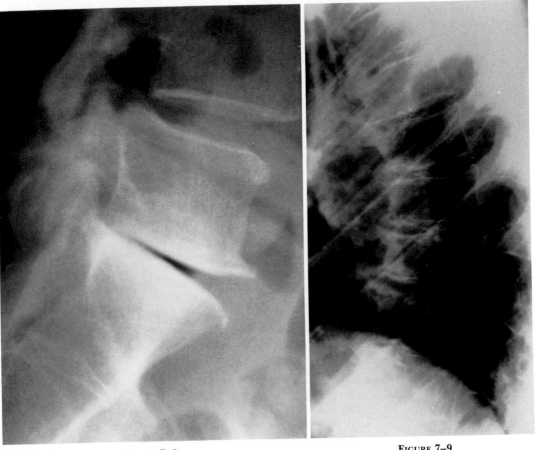

FIGURE 7–8   FIGURE 7–9

FIGURE 7–8. Lateral view of L5-S1. This demonstrates narrowing of the disc space with a vacuum phenomenon. Small marginal osteophytes are present along with subchondral bone repair.

FIGURE 7–9. Lateral view of the thoracic spine in a patient with acromegaly. There is loss of disc height along with osteophyte formation. There is definite increase in the AP diameter of the vertebral body.

When one observes degenerative disc disease at multiple levels without obvious structural abnormality such as rotoscoliosis, one must consider an underlying arthropathy. The most common cause today would be calcium pyrophosphate dihydrate (CPPD) crystal deposition disease, in which one might find calcification in the soft tissue structures near the disc space. **Acromegaly** can be diagnosed when degenerative disc disease is observed in a patient with increase in the AP diameter of his vertebral bodies (Fig. 7–9).

Ochronosis causes degenerative disc disease at all levels manifested by calcification and/or the vacuum phenomenon at all levels in the spine (Fig. 7–10). While there is subchondral sclerosis in the vertebral bodies, there is remarkable absence of osteophyte formation. Sometimes the disc loss is so profound that the spine acts ankylosed.

Observation of extreme or excessive degenerative disc disease should suggest a **neuropathic** spine. There may be dissolution of the disc space, tumbling of one vertebral body into another, reparative bone involving the entire vertebral body, massive osteophyte formation, and bone fragmentation (Fig. 7–11). While once associated with tabes dorsalis, today this change is also observed in diabetic patients.

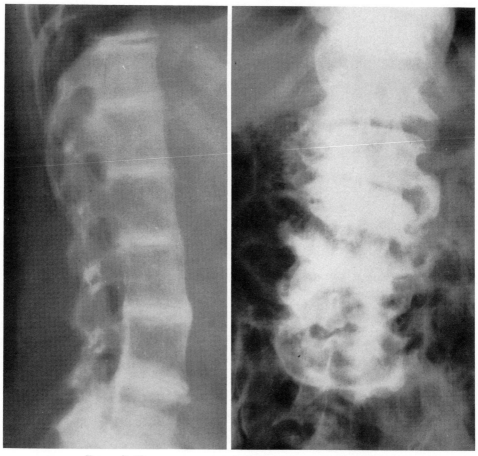

FIGURE 7–10   FIGURE 7–11

FIGURE 7–10. Lateral view of the lumbar spine in a patient with ochronosis. There is total loss of disc space at multiple levels. Calcification and the vacuum phenomenon are present at several levels. There is subchondral sclerosis but absence of osteophyte formation.

FIGURE 7–11. AP view of the lumbar spine in a patient with tabes dorsalis. There is severe loss of disc space, extensive reparative bone, massive osteophyte formation, and some bone fragmentation.

Spondylosis Deformans (Fig. 7–12)

The diagnosis of spondylosis deformans is made when one observes small marginal and/or non-marginal osteophytes surrounding a disc *without* disc space loss or other signs of degenerative disc disease. Spondylosis deformans is thought to be a degeneration of Sharpey's fibers, allowing anterior movement of the disc within the space. This anterior motion is believed to pull on the anterior longitudinal ligament, thus producing the small traction osteophyte. The small marginal osteophyte is produced secondary to the degeneration of Sharpey's fibers.

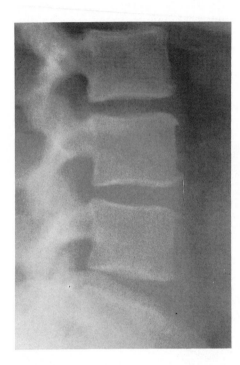

FIGURE 7–12. Lateral view of the lumbar spine in a patient with spondylosis deformans. There is no loss of disc height. There are small marginal osteophytes and non-marginal osteophytes. There is no vertebral body sclerosis.

Ankylosing Spondylitis (Fig. 7–13)

Ankylosing spondylitis produces syndesmophytes. It first ossifies Sharpey's fibers of the anulus fibrosus. It may then ossify the deep layers of the anterior longitudinal ligament. This ossification ascends the spine, from the lumbosacral spine to the cervical spine, in a symmetrical, succinct fashion. The final result is a bamboo spine. It may or may not produce bony ankylosis of the apophyseal joints. The disc spaces are relatively well maintained throughout the spine. Once ankylosed, the disc spaces may become calcified.

Psoriatic and Reiter's Arthritis (Fig. 7–14)

Unlike ankylosing spondylitis, psoriatic and Reiter's involvement of the spine are asymmetrical and exuberant. Although syndesmophytes may be present, more commonly there is production of bridging non-marginal osteophytes. The syndesmophytes and non-marginal osteophytes may be unilateral or bilateral, but in a skip distribution. Again, the apophyseal joints may or may not be ankylosed. The disc spaces tend to be maintained. One cannot distinguish the spine involvement in a patient with psoriasis from that in a patient with Reiter's disease. However, it is unusual for Reiter's disease but fairly common for psoriasis to involve the spine.

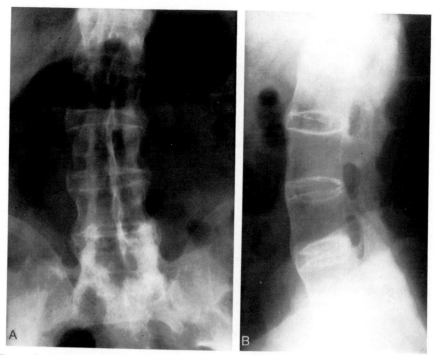

FIGURE 7–13. AP (*A*) and lateral (*B*) views of the lumbar spine in a patient with ankylosing spondylitis. Symmetrical syndesmophytes involve the entire spine. Note the ankylosis of the apophyseal joints. (From Brower AC: The significance of various phytes of the spine. Radiolog 1(15):3, 1978.)

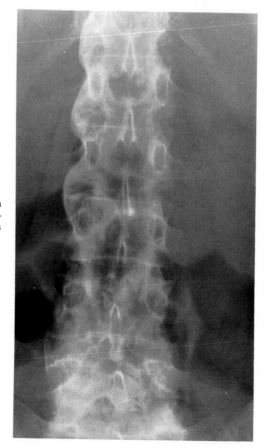

FIGURE 7–14. AP view of the lumbosacral spine in a patient with psoriatic arthritis. There are asymmetrical syndesmophytes and non-marginal osteophytes present.

Diffuse Idiopathic Skeletal Hyperostosis (Figs. 7–15 to 7–18)

The paraspinal phyte is the hallmark of diffuse idiopathic skeletal hyperostosis (DISH). DISH is not an arthropathy. It does not affect joint cartilage or articulating bone. Therefore, the apophyseal joints and the disc spaces are not affected. It is a bone-forming diathesis. It primarily ossifies ligaments and tendons, specifically at their attachments. In the spine, it ossifies the longitudinal ligaments. It is most commonly observed in the thoracic spine as excessive flowing ossification anterior to the vertebral bodies. Unlike ankylosing spondylitis, it does not ossify Sharpey's fibers. Therefore, classically at the disc space levels, the ossification bulges anteriorly, producing a lucent Y- or T-shaped configuration between the ossification and the vertebral end-plates. The diagnosis of DISH is made when this flowing ossification involves four or more contiguous vertebral bodies with their intervening disc spaces (Fig. 7–15). In 10 per cent of the patients with DISH the ossification may be succinct enough to give an appearance similar to that of ankylosing spondylitis (Fig. 7–16). However, usually a lucency can be demonstrated between the ossification of the longitudinal ligament and the vertebral body, which cannot be identified in ankylosing spondylitis. In the cervical spine this ossification may become so extensive as to cause dysphagia (Fig. 7–17). When the lumbar spine is involved, paraspinal phytes are usually seen (Fig. 7–18). However, the lumbar spine may also manifest effusive non-marginal and marginal bridging osteophytes. If the "phytes" in the lumbar spine suggest either DISH or a spondyloarthropathy, one need only observe the sacroiliac joints. These will be normal in DISH and abnormal in the spondyloarthropathies.

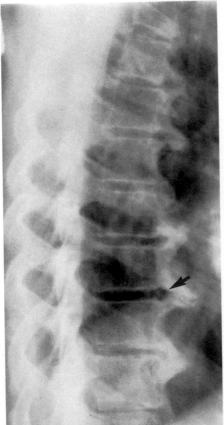

FIGURE 7–15. Lateral view of the thoracic spine in a patient with DISH. Flowing ossification or paraspinal phytes involve most of the thoracic spine. Note the T- or Y-shaped lucency at the disc level demonstrating lack of ossification of the anulus fibrosus (arrow). (From Brower AC: The significance of various phytes of the spine. Radiolog 1(15):3, 1978.)

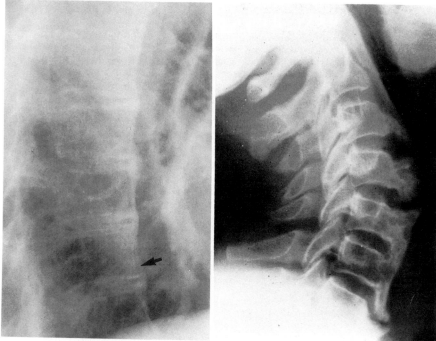

FIGURE 7–16   FIGURE 7–17

FIGURE 7–16. Lateral view of the thoracic spine in a patient with DISH. While this appearance is similar to that of ankylosing spondylitis, a lucency (arrow) separates the following ossification from the vertebral body.

FIGURE 7–17. A lateral view of the cervical spine in a patient with DISH. Note that the disc spaces are maintained and the apophyseal joints are free of disease. There is excessive bone formation anterior to the vertebral bodies.

FIGURE 7–18. Lateral view of the lumbar spine in a patient with DISH. Note the flowing paraspinal phytes.

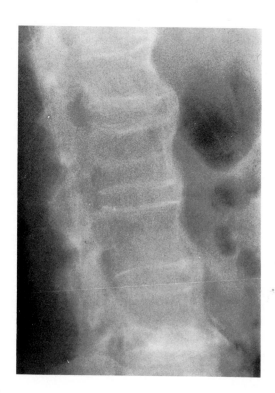

SUGGESTED READINGS

Berens D: Roentgen features of ankylosing spondylitis. Clin Orthop 74:20–33, 1971.

Brower A: The significance of the various phytes of the spine. Radiolog 1(15):3–31, 1978.

Feldman F, Johnson AM, Walter JF: Acute axial neuropathy. Radiology 111:1–16, 1974.

Lang EK, Bessler WT: Roentgenologic features of acromegaly. AJR 6:321–328, 1961.

MacNab I: The traction spur. J Bone Joint Surg 53A:663–670, 1971.

McEwen C, DiTata D, Lingg C, et al.: Ankylosing spondylitis and spondylitis accompanying ulcerative colitis, regional enteritis, psoriasis and Reiter's disease. Arthritis Rheum 14:291–318, 1971.

O'Brien WM, Bunfield WG, Sokoloff L: Studies on the pathogenesis of ochronotic arthropathy. Arthritis Rheum 4:137–152, 1961.

Peterson CC, Silbiger ML: Reiter's syndrome and psoriatic arthritis. Their roentgen spectra and some interesting similarities. AJR 101:860–871, 1967.

Resnick D: Disorders of the axial skeleton which are lesser known, poorly recognized or misunderstood. Bull Rheum Dis 28:932–939, 1977-78.

Resnick D: Osteophytes, syndesmophytes and other "phytes." Postgrad Radiol 1:217–231, 1981.

Resnick D, Niwayama G: Radiographic and pathologic features of spinal involvement in diffuse idiopathic skeletal hyperostosis (DISH). Radiology 119:559–568, 1976.

Sokoloff L: Pathology and pathogenesis of osteoarthritis. Degenerative disease of the spinal column. In Hollander JL (ed): Arthritis and Allied Conditions. Philadelphia, Lea & Febiger, 1966, pp 855–857.

Part II

RADIOGRAPHIC CHANGES OBSERVED IN A SPECIFIC ARTICULAR DISEASE

chapter 8

RHEUMATOID ARTHRITIS

In the practice of rheumatology, rheumatoid arthritis is considered the "everyday" disease. It is a symmetrical arthritis of the appendicular skeleton, sparing the axial skeleton except for the cervical spine. The common radiographic findings are as follows:

1. **Periarticular soft tissue swelling**

2. **Juxta-articular osteoporosis progressing to generalized osteoporosis**

3. **Uniform loss of joint space**

4. **Lack of bone formation**

5. **Marginal erosions progressing to severe erosions of subchondral bone**

6. **Synovial cyst formation**

7. **Subluxations**

8. **Bilateral symmetrical distribution**

9. **Distribution in hands, feet, knees, hips, cervical spine, shoulders, and elbows in decreasing order of frequency**

Not all of these features are present at any one time, and no one abnormality is pathognomonic. However, combinations of many of these findings should lead to the correct diagnosis of rheumatoid arthritis.

THE HANDS

Radiographs of the hands are used by clinicians for two distinct purposes: (1) to help in early diagnosis and (2) to assess disease progression. Therefore, the radiographic changes in the hands and wrists will be described in two separate categories: early changes, observed primarily for diagnosis, and late changes, observed primarily for disease state.

Early Changes

The earliest changes seen radiographically are soft tissue swelling symmetrically around the joints involved and juxta-articular osteoporosis. These changes are non-specific but help to confirm the clinical impression of an inflammatory problem. Erosive disease is an indication of the aggressiveness of the arthropathy. Early erosions are subtle radiographically and must be specifically looked for. The first erosive changes occur before there is loss of joint space. Erosions occur in the "bare" areas of bone, or the bone within the joint space capsule which is not covered by articular cartilage. Radiographically one loses the continuity of the white cortical line. On the PA view, this is best observed in the heads of the metacarpals (Fig. 8–1) and at the margins of the PIP joints (Fig. 8–2). However, erosions are often first observed on the radial aspect of the base of the proximal phalanges. These changes are best imaged on the Norgaard, or semisupinated oblique, view of the hands (Fig. 8–3) (see Chapter 1).

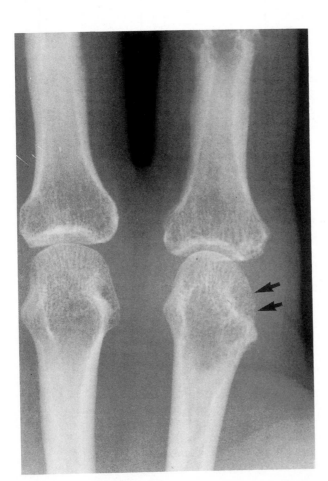

FIGURE 8–1. Metacarpophalangeal joint: early changes. Loss of white cortical line (arrows) representing erosion of bare area.

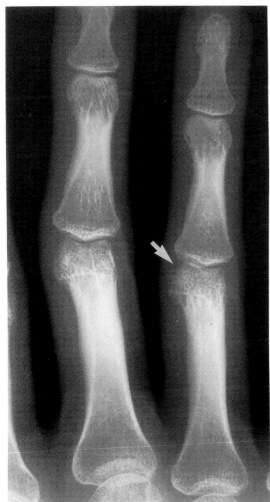

FIGURE 8–2. Proximal interphalangeal joint of a finger: early changes. Marginal erosion demonstrated (arrow).

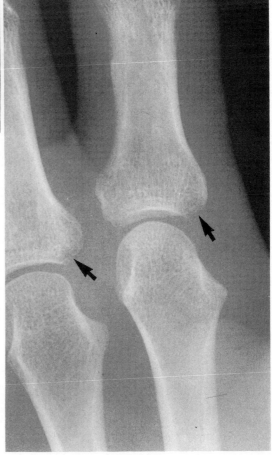

FIGURE 8–3. Metacarpophalangeal joint: early changes. Norgaard projection demonstrating erosion of the radial aspect at the base of the proximal phalanx (arrows).

In the wrist, early erosions must be looked for in specific locations. They commonly occur at the waist of the navicular, the waist of the capitate, the articulation of the hamate with the base of the fifth metacarpal, the articulation of the first metacarpal with the greater multangular, the radial styloid, and the ulnar styloid. These can all be imaged on the PA view (Fig. 8–4A and B). The Norgaard view profiles the pisiform and triquetrium and often demonstrates erosive changes between these two bones before erosions are seen on the ulnar styloid (Fig. 8–4C).

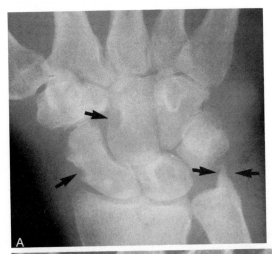

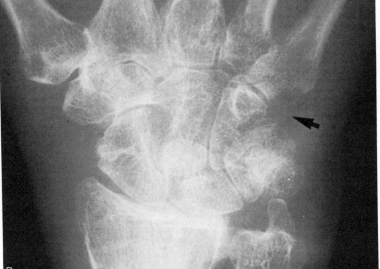

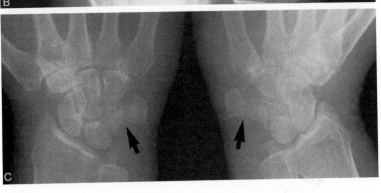

FIGURE 8–4. *A*, PA view of the wrist demonstrating early changes. Erosion of the waist of the navicular, the waist of the capitate, and the ulnar styloid (arrows). Note that mineralization is normal and joint spaces are maintained. *B*, PA view of the wrist showing juxta-articular osteoporosis and mild loss of joint spaces in a pancarpal distribution. Note erosion of the hamate as it articulates with the base of the 5th metacarpal (arrow). *C*, Norgaard view of the wrist demonstrating erosive changes between the triquetrium and the pisiform bilaterally (arrows). Note that the ulnar styloid is intact. (*C* from Kantor S, Brower AC: Radiographic assessment. *In* Rothermich N, Whisler R: Rheumatoid Arthritis. Orlando, FL, Grune & Stratton, Inc, 1985, p 57.)

Late Changes

In the hand, the MCP's and/or the PIP's are uniformly involved. In the wrist, all the carpals are affected as a unit. As the disease progresses, the cartilage and apparent joint space are lost uniformly (Fig. 8–5). As the cartilage is lost, the soft tissue swelling caused by a rheumatoid synovitis decreases. Juxta-articular osteoporosis progresses to diffuse osteoporosis. The subtle marginal erosions continue to progress, involving more and more of the articular surface to become large subchondral erosions (Fig. 8–6). Subluxations occur at the MCP joints with the proximal phalanges subluxating ulnarly and palmarly in relationship to the metacarpal heads (Fig. 8–7). Swan-neck and boutonniere deformities develop in the distal phalanges. Although the subluxations occur secondary to inflammation of the tendons and ligaments surrounding the joint, erosive disease is usually present when the subluxations occur.

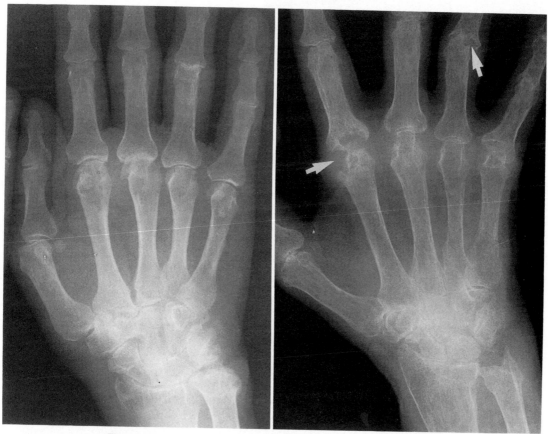

FIGURE 8–5

FIGURE 8–6

FIGURE 8–5. PA view of the hand in advanced stages of rheumatoid arthritis. Diffuse osteoporosis is apparent. Note the uniform involvement of PIP joints, MCP joints, and carpal bones as a unit. (From Kantor S, Brower AC: Radiographic assessment. *In* Rothermich N, Whisler R: Rheumatoid Arthritis. Orlando, FL, Grune & Stratton, Inc, 1985, p 57.)

FIGURE 8–6. PA view of the hand in late stages of rheumatoid arthritis. Note the profound osteoporosis. There is PIP, MCP, and pancarpal involvement. Note the large subchondral erosion of the 2nd MCP and the 4th PIP joints (arrows). (From Brower AC: The radiologic approach to arthritis. Med Clin North Am 68:1593, 1984.)

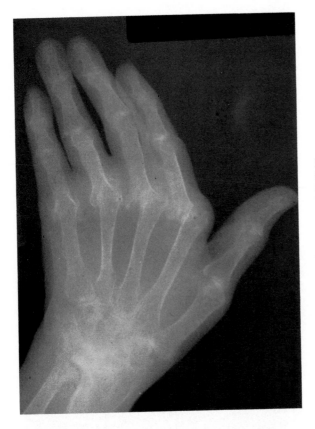

FIGURE 8–7. PA view of the hand demonstrating late changes of rheumatoid arthritis. Note the diffuse osteoporosis. There is actual soft tissue atrophy. There is involvement of the PIP's, the MCP's, and the carpals as a unit. There is severe erosion, so that normal bone contour is not present. The proximal phalanges are subluxating ulnarly and palmarly in relationship to the metacarpal heads.

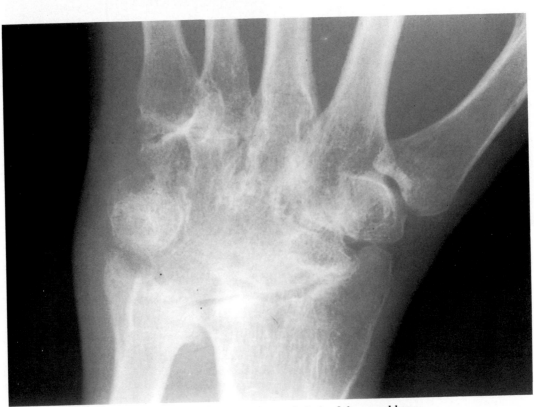

FIGURE 8–8. PA view of the wrist demonstrating bone ankylosis of the carpal bones.

In the late stages of the disease there is actually soft tissue atrophy. Diffuse osteoporosis is present. Subcutaneous rheumatoid nodules may develop in 25 per cent of the patients. The nodules themselves do not cause bone destruction. There is lack of recognizable joint spaces (Fig. 8–7). Bone ankylosis of the carpals may occur (Fig. 8–8). Although there may be fibrous ankylosis of the phalanges, there should be no radiographic evidence of bone ankylosis distal to the carpals unless there has been surgical fusion. Despite extensive involvement of the PIP's and MCP's, the DIP's are usually spared. If there are erosive changes involving the DIP's, a second arthropathy such as erosive osteoarthritis should be considered. The hand may eventually become an arthritis mutilans (Fig. 8–9).

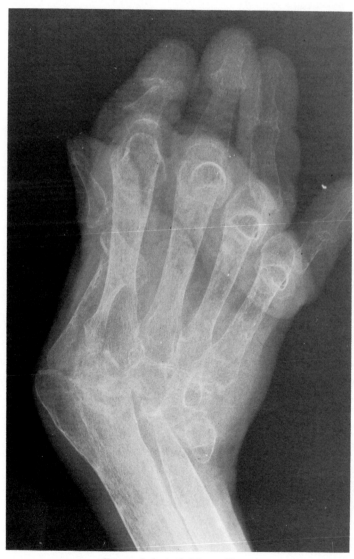

FIGURE 8–9. Arthritis mutilans.

THE FEET

The feet are involved in 80 to 90 per cent of patients. Some observers state that in 10 to 20 per cent of patients, the feet are involved before the hands. However, generally the changes in the feet accompany or lag somewhat behind the changes in the hands.

The radiographic changes in the feet are evaluated through a PA and a lateral view. Early involvement of the feet again shows a juxta-articular osteoporosis and erosion of the bare areas on the heads of the metatarsals. The first erosive change is seen on the lateral aspect of the head of the fifth metatarsal (Fig. 8–10). There is loss of the white cortical line. The other metatarsal heads are eroded primarily medially and later laterally (Fig. 8–11). As the disease progresses, there are uniform loss of the cartilage in the MTP joints, progressive erosive changes, and subluxations of the proximal phalanges in a fibular direction in relationship to the metatarsals (Fig. 8–12). The metatarsal heads also subluxate in a plantar direction. There are dorsiflexion deformities of the PIP joints and a hallux valgus deformity of the big toe.

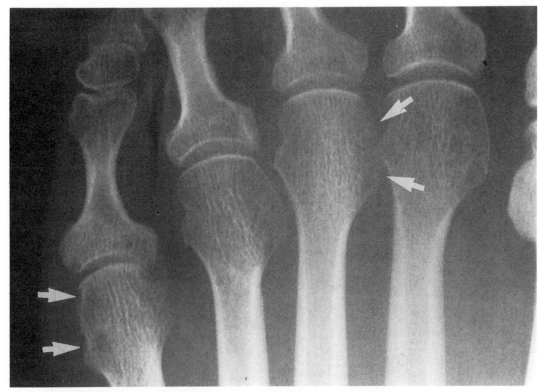

FIGURE 8–10. PA view of the metatarsophalangeal joints: early changes. Erosion of the lateral aspect of the head of the 5th metatarsal and the medial aspect of the head of the 3rd metatarsal (arrows).

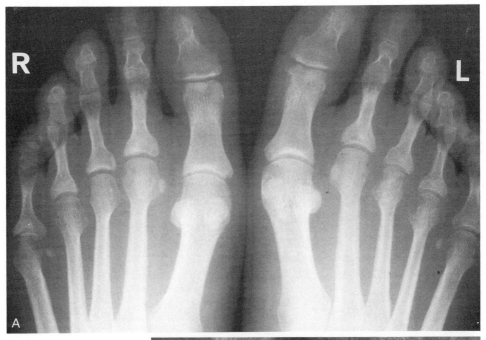

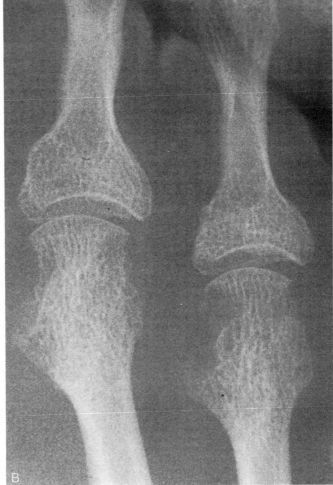

FIGURE 8–11. *A*, AP view of both fore-feet. *B*, Magnified view of the 3rd and 4th MTP joints of the left foot: early changes. Joint spaces are maintained. Erosive changes of the medial aspect of metatarsal heads are larger than those on the lateral aspect.

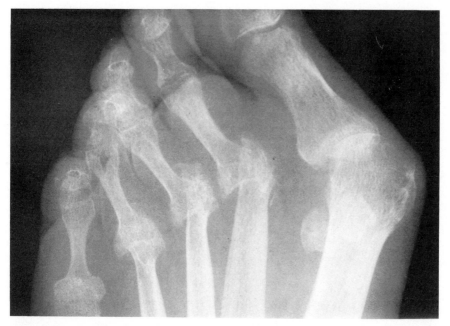

FIGURE 8–12. AP view of the forefoot: late changes of rheumatoid arthritis. Note osteoporosis, severe erosive changes involving the heads of the metatarsals, hallux valgus deformity, and fibular subluxation of the proximal phalanges in relationship to the metatarsal heads.

Like the carpal bones in the wrist, the tarsal bones in the foot are involved as a unit, with uniform joint space loss (Fig. 8–13). Bone ankylosis may occur in the tarsals but not distal to the tarsals (Fig. 8–14). Erosive changes may be present in the calcaneus at the attachment of the plantar aponeurosis and/or the attachment of the Achilles tendon (Fig. 8–15).

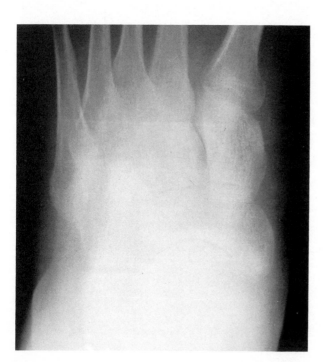

FIGURE 8–13. AP view of the mid-foot demonstrating uniform cartilage loss between all the tarsal bones.

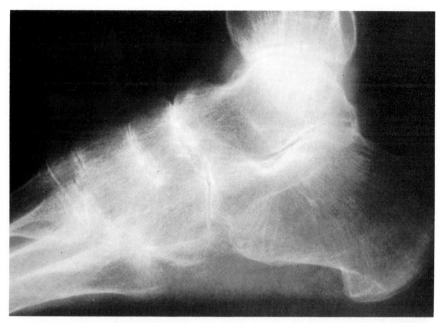

FIGURE 8–14. Lateral view of the mid and hind foot showing narrowing of all the tarsal joint spaces, severe osteoporosis, and bone ankylosis between the navicular, cuboid, and cuneiforms.

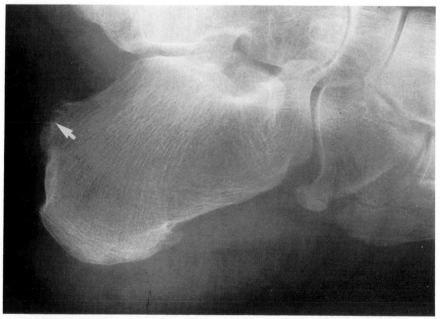

FIGURE 8–15. Lateral view of the calcaneus showing erosion at the attachment of the Achilles tendon (arrow).

THE HIPS

The hip joint is involved less frequently than the knee. It is affected in 50 per cent of patients. There is uniform loss of the cartilage and therefore axial migration of the femoral head within the acetabulum (Fig. 8–16). As the cartilage is lost, the head continues to move in an axial or a superomedial direction (Fig. 8–17). Bone is eroded away on the joint side of the acetabulum and laid down on the pelvic side, producing a protrusion of the acetabulum. Both hips are affected in a symmetrical fashion.

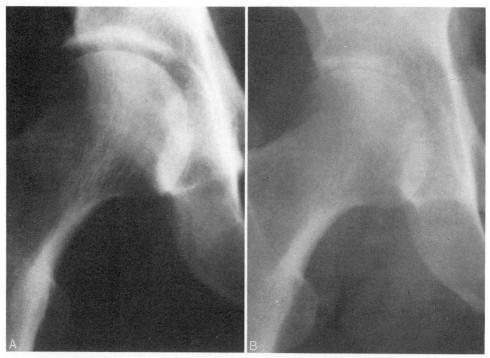

FIGURE 8–16. Rheumatoid hip: early changes. *A,* Normal hip. *B,* Same hip one year later showing uniform cartilage loss with axial migration.

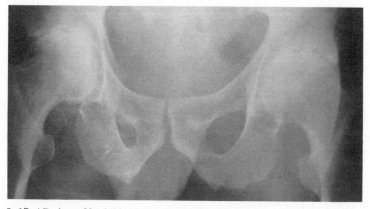

FIGURE 8–17. AP view of both hips in a patient with rheumatoid arthritis. There is bilateral axial migration. There is minimal erosive disease. There is no evidence of osteophyte formation or reparative bone.

With cartilage loss, there are varying degrees of erosion and synovial cyst formation (Fig. 8–18). The changes in the femoral head also may be complicated by osteonecrosis secondary to steroid therapy. However, despite these changes and despite total loss of cartilage, the adjacent bone does not respond with reparative phenomena such as osteophytes or subchondral bone formation. Therefore, the typical rheumatoid pelvis shows bilateral symmetrical involvement of the hips with acetabuli protrusio, osteoporosis, and noticeable absence of reparative bone and osteophyte formation (Fig. 8–19).

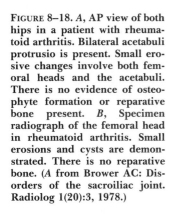

FIGURE 8–18. *A*, AP view of both hips in a patient with rheumatoid arthritis. Bilateral acetabuli protrusio is present. Small erosive changes involve both femoral heads and the acetabuli. There is no evidence of osteophyte formation or reparative bone present. *B*, Specimen radiograph of the femoral head in rheumatoid arthritis. Small erosions and cysts are demonstrated. There is no reparative bone. (*A* from Brower AC: Disorders of the sacroiliac joint. Radiolog 1(20):3, 1978.)

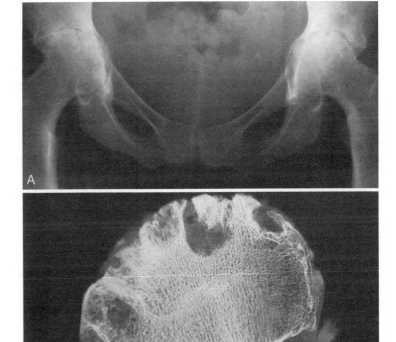

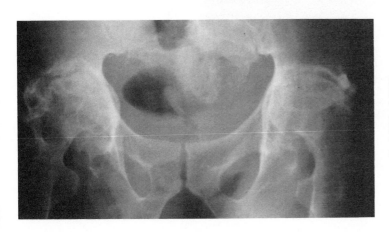

FIGURE 8–19. AP view of both hips in severe rheumatoid arthritis. There is severe bilateral acetabuli protrusio. Note that the protrusion is in a superomedial direction. There is severe osteoporosis. There is no evidence of reparative bone.

THE SACROILIAC JOINTS

Involvement of the sacroiliac (SI) joints in rheumatoid arthritis is relatively insignificant. It occurs late in the patient's disease, if at all, and the patient and physician are more concerned about the involvement of the hands, feet, hips, or knees. Involvement of the SI joints is seen as a uniform narrowing of the joint space without evidence of bone repair or osteophyte formation (Fig. 8–20). While erosive change can occur, it is never extensive enough to produce the apparent widening that one sees in the spondyloarthropathies. Bone ankylosis can occur, but only of the true synovial aspect of the SI joint (Fig. 8–21).

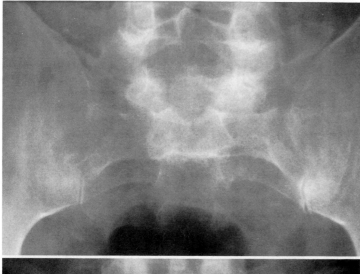

FIGURE 8–20. AP view of SI joints. There is bilateral symmetrical narrowing of the SI joints. There is generalized osteoporosis. There is no erosive disease and minimal bone repair.

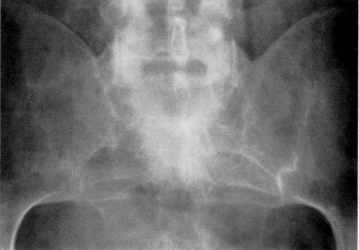

FIGURE 8–21. AP view of the SI joints showing bone ankylosis of the synovial aspect of the joint.

THE KNEES

The knees are involved in 80 per cent of patients. They are involved bilaterally and symmetrically. Radiographically, the knees must be evaluated with a standing AP view and a flexed lateral view to assess cartilage loss and alignment accurately. There is uniform loss of the cartilage or loss of the cartilage in all three compartments of the knee: the medial, the lateral, and the patellofemoral. Despite even severe loss of cartilage, there is little, if any, reparative response; there is a noticeable lack of subchondral bone and osteophyte formation (Fig. 8–22). Marginal erosions may occur but are not as prominent a part of the radiographic picture as they are in the hands. However, intraosseous synovial cysts may play a significant role. Such a cyst is produced by synovium breaking through the cartilage and protruding into the bone. A ball-valve effect on the synovial fluid within the cyst causes enlargement of the cyst. Large cysts are called "geods." Sometimes these geods are mistaken for a bone neoplasm (Fig. 8–23). However, the presence of uniform joint space narrowing and adjacent smaller cysts should indicate the correct diagnosis.

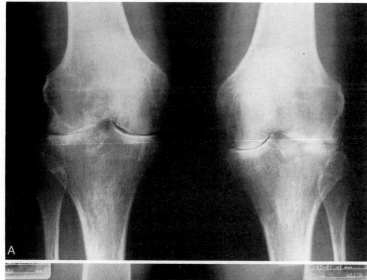

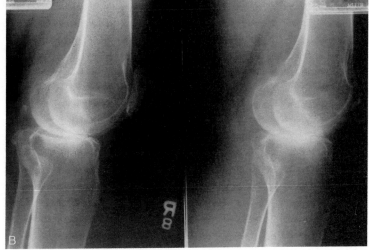

FIGURE 8–22. *A*, AP standing view and (*B*) lateral view of both knees demonstrating cartilage loss of the medial, lateral, and patellofemoral compartments. There is generalized osteoporosis present. Erosive disease is not a prominent feature. There is no evidence of bone repair. (*A* from Kantor S, Brower AC: Radiographic assessment. *In* Rothermich N, Whisler R: Rheumatoid Arthritis. Orlando, FL, Grune & Stratton, Inc, 1985, p 57.)

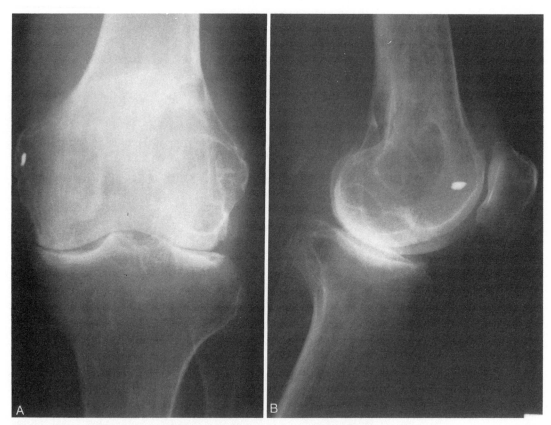

FIGURE 8–23. AP (*A*) and lateral (*B*) views of the knee in a patient with rheumatoid arthritis. A large synovial cyst involves the lateral femoral condyle and resembles a giant cell tumor. However, there is narrowing of the medial, lateral, and patellofemoral compartments. There is also a synovial cyst involving the adjacent tibial plateau. There is generalized osteoporosis. These related findings lead to the diagnosis of a rheumatoid "geod" rather than a giant cell tumor. (From Kantor S, Brower AC: Radiographic assessment. *In* Rothermich N, Whisler R: Rheumatoid Arthritis. Orlando, FL, Grune & Stratton, Inc, 1985, p 57.)

A Baker's cyst, or synovial cyst extending into the soft tissues, is a frequent occurrence in rheumatoid arthritis. It extends posteriorly and may be directed inferiorly or superiorly in the soft tissues in the back of the knee. Ultrasound is often used to confirm the presence of a cyst. Rupture of a cyst with extravasation of cyst material into the surrounding muscle may cause symptoms similar to those of thrombophlebitis. An arthrogram showing extravasation of contrast material from the cyst permits the appropriate diagnosis (Fig. 8–24). However, it must be remembered that a Baker's cyst that has not ruptured can cause increased pressure on the deep venous system, producing a true thrombophlebitis.

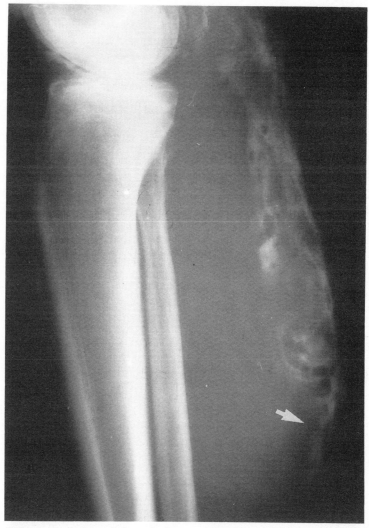

FIGURE 8–24. Lateral view of the soft tissues posterior to the knee and tibia. Contrast material has been instilled into a Baker's cyst and shows rupture of the Baker's cyst inferiorly (arrow).

THE ANKLES

The ankle is involved less frequently than the hand, foot, and knee. When involved, the ankles show bilateral and symmetrical involvement. There is uniform loss of the cartilage in the ankle joint with lack of reparative response (Fig. 8–25). Erosive changes do not play a prominant role. Synovial cysts may be present. A unique feature of ankle involvement is periosteal reaction that may occur along the posterior shaft of the tibia. This may be just a manifestation of the patient's underlying disease. However, one must be careful to distinguish this periostitis from that occurring with a secondary stress fracture or osteomyelitis (Fig. 8–26).

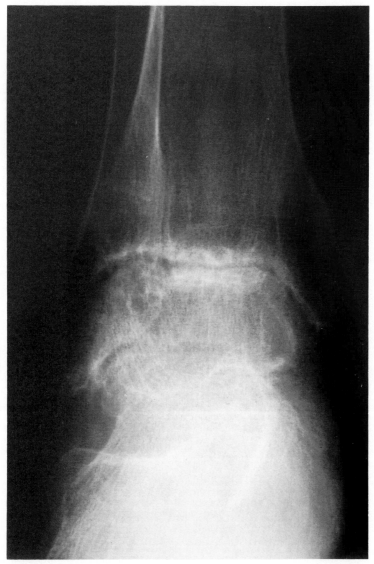

FIGURE 8–25. AP view of the ankle in rheumatoid arthritis showing uniform narrowing of the joint space with severe osteoporosis of the surrounding bone structures.

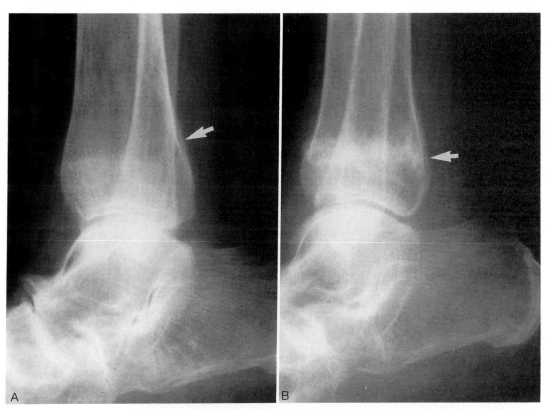

FIGURE 8–26. Lateral view of the ankle in rheumatoid arthritis. *A*, Generalized osteoporosis. Narrowing of the tarsal joints is visualized. There is a fine linear periosteal reaction posteriorly on the inferior aspect of the tibia (arrow). *B*, Same ankle 10 days later demonstrating a stress fracture (arrow) of the distal tibia as the cause of the periosteal response.

THE SHOULDERS

Sixty per cent of patients ultimately have involvement of the shoulders. Radiographically, there is uniform narrowing of all compartments of the shoulder joint: the glenohumeral, the acromiohumeral, and the acromioclavicular joint. The humeral head therefore migrates proximally and superiorly in relationship to the glenoid (Fig. 8–27). There is usually an associated rotator cuff tear that allows the narrowing between the humerus and acromion. One may identify an actual erosion at the rotator cuff attachment (Fig. 8–28). Generalized osteoporosis is present. There is no evidence of bone repair or osteophyte formation. A synovial cyst may be present in the humeral head and may be mistaken for a chondroblastoma; however, the joint space narrowing should preclude this diagnosis. There will be erosion of the distal end of the clavicle. Likewise, there may be erosion of the proximal end of the clavicle, as the sternoclavicular joint is also a synovial joint (Fig. 8–29).

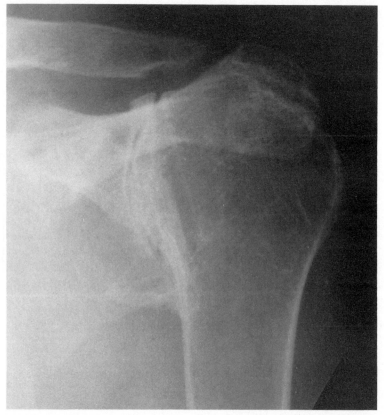

FIGURE 8–27. AP view of the shoulder showing generalized osteoporosis. The humeral head has migrated proximally and superiorly owing to loss of cartilage in the glenohumeral joint and the acromiohumeral joint. There is erosion of the distal end of the clavicle.

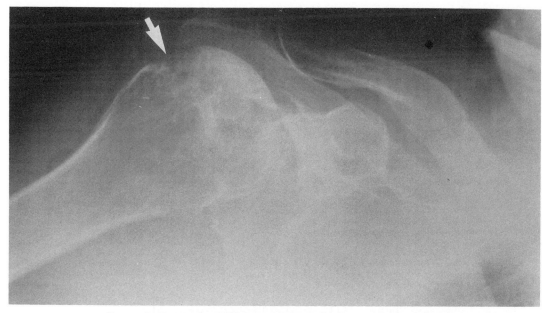

FIGURE 8–28. AP view of the shoulder showing generalized osteoporosis. Erosive changes (arrow) are demonstrated in the humeral head.

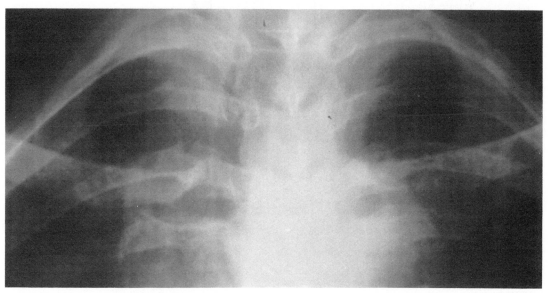

FIGURE 8–29. Erosive changes of the proximal end of the clavicle. (From Kantor S, Brower AC: Radiographic assessment. *In* Rothermich N, Whisler R: Rheumatoid Arthritis. Orlando, FL, Grune & Stratton, Inc, 1985, p 57.)

THE ELBOWS

The elbow is involved in 34 per cent of patients. When involved, the elbows show bilateral symmetrical involvement with uniform loss of the joint space. Generalized osteoporosis is present, and there is distinct lack of reparative bone and osteophyte formation (Fig. 8–30). The elbow joint may be so destroyed as to give the appearance of widening of the joint space (Fig. 8–31). Synovial cysts may occur around the elbow as well (Fig. 8–32).

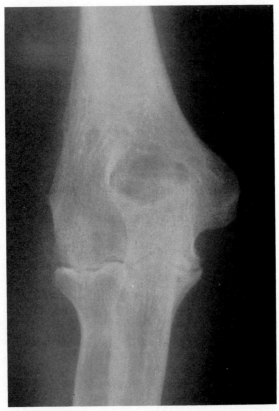

FIGURE 8–30. AP view of the elbow showing uniform joint space loss between the radius and the humerus as well as between the ulna and the humerus. There is generalized osteoporosis. There is no evidence of reparative bone.

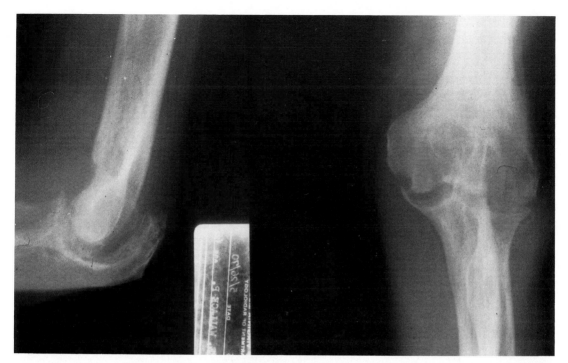

FIGURE 8–31. Lateral and AP views of the elbow showing such severe joint space loss as to give a widened appearance to the joint. There is severe osteoporosis present.

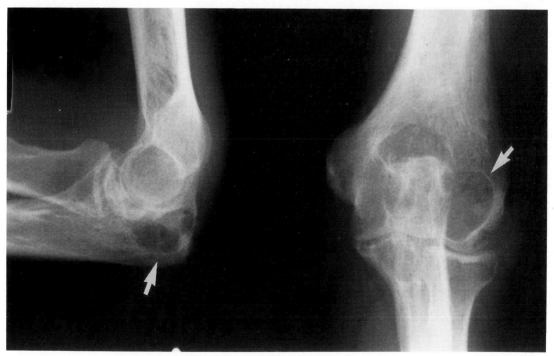

FIGURE 8–32. Lateral and AP views of the elbow. There are uniform joint space loss, osteoporosis, and synovial cysts (arrows).

THE SPINE

The thoracic and lumbar areas of the spine are usually not significantly involved in rheumatoid arthritis. However, the cervical spine is involved in approximately 50 per cent of individuals with rheumatoid arthritis. The most common abnormality seen in the cervical spine is atlanto-axial disease. The most frequent radiographic finding is laxity of the transverse ligament that holds the odontoid to the atlas. This laxity becomes apparent in the flexed lateral view of the cervical spine; unless the radiograph is taken in this position this abnormality will be missed (Fig. 8–33). If every patient with rheumatoid arthritis had their cervical spine radiographed in the flexed position, 33 per cent would have this abnormality demonstrated. This laxity may become so severe as to require posterior fusion. It is believed that a gap of 8 mm or more between the odontoid and atlas requires surgical intervention (Fig. 8–34).

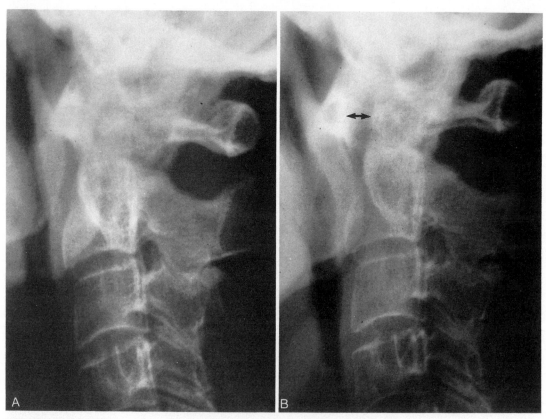

FIGURE 8–33. Lateral views of the C1-C2 area in rheumatoid arthritis. *A*, Film was obtained in neutral position and shows no significant abnormality. *B*, Film taken with the neck in a flexed position demonstrates increased distance between the atlas and odontoid (arrows). This demonstrates nicely the laxity of the transverse ligament.

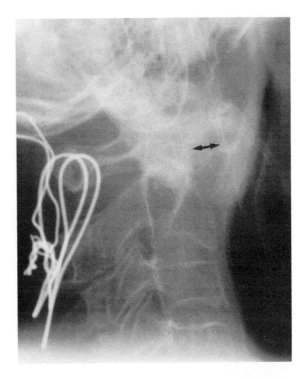

FIGURE 8–34. Lateral view of the upper cervical spine in late rheumatoid arthritis. Posterior fusion has been undertaken. The distance between the atlas and the odontoid (arrow) was greater than 8 mm.

A more severe manifestation of atlanto-axial disease is vertical subluxation, or upward translocation of the dens (Fig. 8–35). One must assess the tip of the odontoid in relationship to the base of the skull. Erosion of the tip of the odontoid may serve as protection in patients with this malalignment. However, erosion of the odontoid is not as common as subluxation of the atlanto-axial joint.

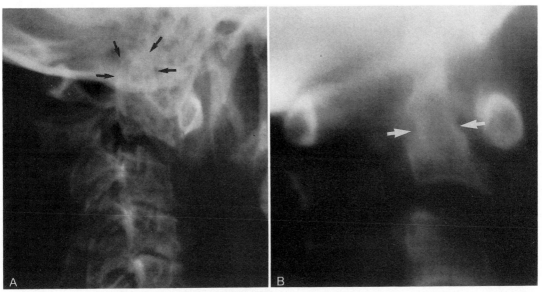

FIGURE 8–35. Lateral views of the upper cervical spine. *A*, Plain film shows upward translocation of the dens (arrows outline the top of the dens). *B*, Tomogram confirms this and shows erosion (arrows below the odontoid).

The apophyseal joints are commonly involved with erosive disease. Early erosive changes may be seen only on the flexed lateral view of the spine (Fig. 8–36). Progressive involvement of the apophyseal joints leads to osteoporosis, disc space loss, and subluxations at multiple levels (Fig. 8–37). Very rarely the apophyseal joints may ankylose.

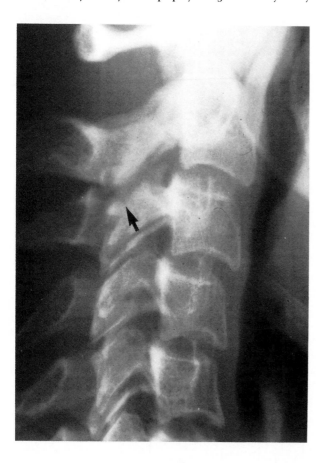

FIGURE 8–36. Flexed lateral view of the cervical spine. Erosive changes (arrow) are seen at the apophyseal joint of C2-C3.

FIGURE 8–37. Lateral view of the cervical spine demonstrating late changes of rheumatoid arthritis. There is severe osteoporosis. There are severe subaxial subluxations with loss of the disc space at C3-C4 and C4-C5. (From Kantor S, Brower AC: Radiographic assessment. In Rothermich N, Whisler R: Rheumatoid Arthritis. Orlando, FL, Grune & Stratton, Inc, 1985, p. 57.)

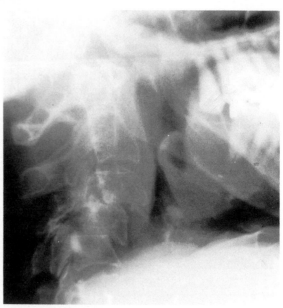

Disc destruction and adjacent vertebral body destruction can occur from a synovitis extending from the joint of Luschka (Fig. 8–38). This must not be mistaken for infection. Despite the high percentage of patients with radiographically detectable cervical spine disease, only a small percentage eventually develop cervical myelopathy. Magnetic resonance imaging may be used to evaluate spinal cord involvement.

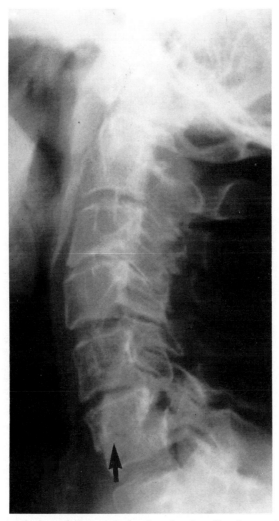

FIGURE 8–38. Lateral view of the cervical spine showing disc destruction and adjacent vertebral body destruction at C6-C7 (arrow). This is caused by a synovitis extending from the joint of Luschka.

THE TEMPOROMANDIBULAR JOINT

The temporomandibular joint (TMJ) is often the forgotten joint in rheumatoid arthritis, but 80 per cent of patients have TMJ symptoms. Osteoporosis, joint space narrowing, decreased range of motion, erosions of the condyle, and flattening of the glenoid fossa are the radiographic changes (Fig. 8–39). These are best demonstrated through conventional tomography, although magnetic resonance imaging may become the modality of choice. Erosive disease may occur in the TMJ without significant erosive disease elsewhere in the body.

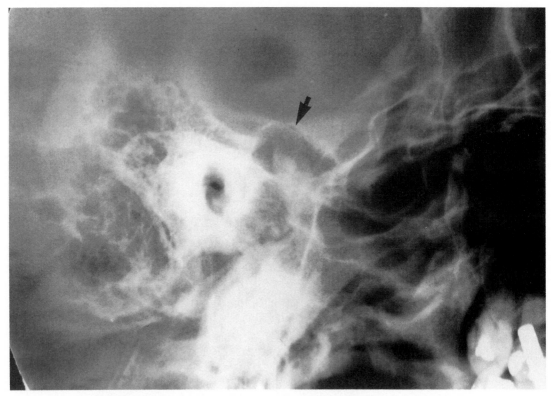

FIGURE 8–39. Lateral view of the temporomandibular joint in the closed position. There are osteoporosis, joint space loss, and severe erosion of the condyle (arrow).

SUMMARY

Rheumatoid arthritis is a common arthropathy with characteristic radiographic joint changes and distribution. Its hallmarks are symmetry, osteoporosis, uniform cartilage loss, erosions, and lack of bone response or proliferation.

SUGGESTED READINGS

Berens DL, Lockie LM, Lin RK, Norcross BM: Roentgen changes in early rheumatoid arthritis. Wrist-Hands-Feet. Radiology 82:645, 1964.

Brewerton DA: Hand deformities in rheumatoid disease. Ann Rheum Dis 16:183, 1957.

Calabro JJ: A critical evaluation of the diagnostic features of the feet in rheumatoid arthritis. Arthritis Rheum 5:19, 1962.

Chalmers IM, Blair GS: Rheumatoid arthritis of the temporomandibular joint: A clinical and radiologic study using circular tomography. Q J Med 42:369, 1973.

Good AE: Rheumatoid arthritis, Baker's cyst and thrombophlebitis. Arthritis Rheum 7:56, 1964.

Hastings DE, Parker SM: Protrusio acetabuli in rheumatoid arthritis. Clin Orthop Rel Res 108:76, 1975.

Kalliomaki JL, Viitanen S-M, Virtama P: Radiological findings of sternoclavicular joints in rheumatoid arthritis. Acta Rheumatol Scand 14:233, 1968.

Kirkup JR: Ankle and tarsal joints in rheumatoid arthritis. Scand J Rheumatol 3:50, 1974.

Komusi T, Munro T, Harth M: Radiologic review: The rheumatoid cervical spine. Semin Arthritis Rheum 14:187–195, 1985.

Magyar E, Talerman A, Feher M, Wouters HW: The pathogenesis of the subchondral pseudocysts in rheumatoid arthritis. Clin Orthop 100:341, 1974.

Martel W: Diagnostic radiology in the rheumatic diseases. *In* Kelley WN, Harris ED, Ruddy S, et al. (eds.): Textbook of Rheumatology. Philadelphia, W. B. Saunders Company, 1981.

Martel W, Duff IF: Pelvo-spondylitis in rheumatoid arthritis. Radiology 77:744, 1961.

Martel W, Hayes JT, Duff IF: The pattern of bone erosion in the hand and wrist in rheumatoid arthritis. Radiology 84:204, 1965.

Norgaard F: Earliest roentgenological changes in polyarthritis of the rheumatoid type: Rheumatoid arthritis. Radiology 85:325, 1965.

Park W, O'Neill M, McCall IW: The radiology of rheumatoid involvement of the cervical spine. Skeletal Radiol 4:1–7, 1979.

Resnick D: Patterns of migration of the femoral head in osteoarthritis of the hip: Roentgenographic-pathologic correlation and comparison with rheumatoid arthritis. AJR 124:62, 1975.

Resnick D: Rheumatoid arthritis of the wrist: The compartmental approach. Med Radiogr Photogr 52:50–88, 1976.

Resnick D, Niwayama G: Rheumatoid arthritis and related diseases. *In* Resnick D, Niwayama G (eds.): Diagnosis of Bone and Joint Disorders. Vol 2. Philadelphia, W. B. Saunders Company, 1981.

Sbarbaro JL: The rheumatoid shoulder. Orthop Clin North Am 6:593, 1975.

Weissman BNW, Aliabadi P, Weinfield LS: Prognostic features of atlanto-axial subluxation in rheumatoid arthritis patients. Radiology 144:745–751, 1982.

Weston WJ: The synovial changes at the elbow in rheumatoid arthritis. Australas Radiol 15:170, 1971.

chapter 9

PSORIATIC ARTHRITIS

For years psoriatic arthritis was considered part of the spectrum of rheumatoid arthritis. The classification of psoriatic arthritis as a "rheumatoid variant" persists today. However, the radiographic manifestations, along with clinical and laboratory data, establish psoriatic arthritis as a separate and distinct articular disorder. Psoriatic arthritis may coincide with or antedate the appearance of skin disease. In these patients, the radiographic examination becomes the determinate diagnostic study. The distinguishing radiographic features are as follows:

1. Fusiform soft tissue swelling

2. Maintenance of normal mineralization

3. Dramatic joint space loss

4. Bone proliferation

5. "Pencil-in-cup" erosions

6. Bilateral asymmetrical distribution

7. Distribution primarily in hands, feet, sacroiliac joints, and spine in decreasing order of frequency

While psoriatic arthritis differs from rheumatoid arthritis radiographically in many ways, the most significant difference is the presence of bone proliferation.

THE HANDS

The hands are most commonly involved in psoriatic arthritis. While there may be periarticular soft tissue swelling, there is often soft tissue edema beyond the joint, causing swelling of the entire digit. This swelling is described as "sausage-like" or resembling a "cocktail hotdog" (Fig. 9–1). Juxta-articular osteoporosis may occur in the early phases of the disease; however, it is transient. Normal mineralization is usually maintained even in the presence of severe erosive disease. Erosions occur initially at the margins of the joint but with time progress to involve the central area (Fig. 9–2). The erosion may become so extensive, destroying so much of the underlying bone, that the joint space may actually appear to be widened. The ends of the bones may become pointed, appearing as if destroyed by a pencil sharpener. The bone articulating with the pointed bone may become saucerized through erosion, producing the classic "pencil-in-cup" or "cup-and-saucer" appearance (Fig. 9–3).

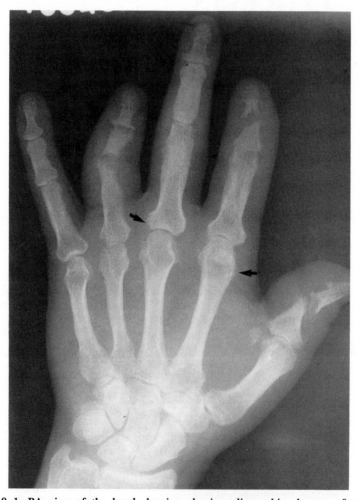

FIGURE 9–1. PA view of the hand showing classic radiographic changes of psoriatic arthritis: "sausage-like" swelling of the 1st, 2nd, and 4th digits; normal mineralization; severe erosive changes creating the appearance of widened joint spaces of the 1st IP, the 2nd DIP, and the 4th PIP joints; solid periosteal new bone added to the proximal phalanx of 2nd digit and the middle and proximal phalanges of 3rd digit, widening the shafts; fluffy new bone apposition adjacent to erosive changes (arrows). (From Brower AC: The radiographic features of psoriatic arthritis. *In* Gerber L, Espinoza L (eds): Psoriatic Arthritis. Orlando, FL, Grune & Stratton, Inc, 1985, p 125.)

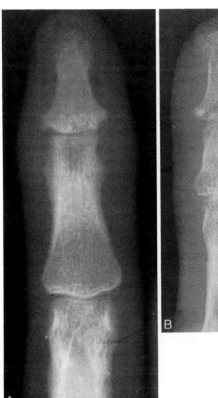
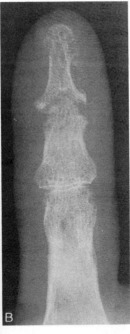

FIGURE 9–2. *A,* Marginal erosions of the DIP joint. *B,* Marginal erosions have progressed to involve the central area of the DIP joint. (From Brower AC: The radiographic features of psoriatic arthritis. *In* Gerber L, Espinoza L (eds): Psoriatic Arthritis. Orlando, FL, Grune & Stratton, Inc, 1985, p 125.)

FIGURE 9–3. Severe erosion of the DIP joint with pencil pointing of the middle phalanx and saucerization of the distal phalanx. Note the widened joint space.

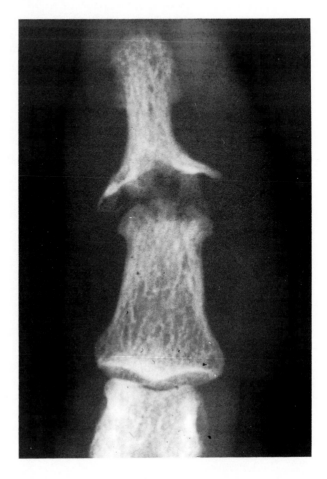

Bone proliferation is one of the most important features of psoriatic arthritis and is almost always present in some form. Bone proliferation takes place in four areas: adjacent to erosions, along shafts, across joints, and at tendinous and ligamentous insertions. The bone proliferation adjacent to erosive changes is observed as irregular excrescences with a spiculated, frayed, or fluffy appearance. With time these excrescences become well-defined bone (Fig. 9–4). Bone proliferation may be observed along shafts as a periostitis (Fig. 9–5). Initially it is exuberant and fluffy in appearance. Eventually it becomes solid new bone along the shaft of the phalanx, causing the widened appearance to the phalanx (Fig. 9–1). Bone ankylosis across a joint is a common occurrence in DIP and PIP joints (Fig. 9–6). Bone proliferation occurring at tendinous and ligamentous insertions in the hand and wrist will be seen as a continuation of the periosteal response.

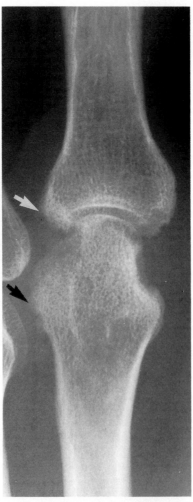

FIGURE 9–4. Bone proliferation (arrows) adjacent to erosive changes. Some excrescences are well defined, whereas others are more irregular in appearance.

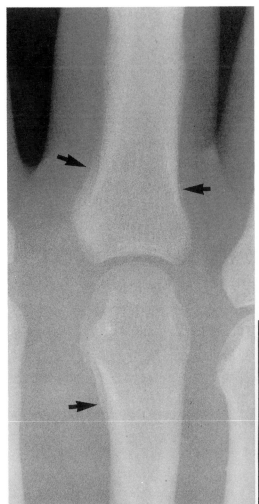

FIGURE 9–5. Periostitis (arrows) along the shafts of bones.

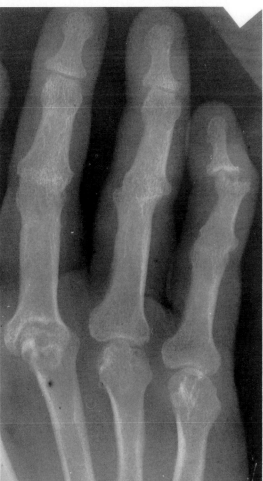

FIGURE 9–6. Bone ankylosis of the 3rd, 4th, and 5th PIP joints.

In the hand, psoriatic arthritis classically involves the DIP and PIP joints, with relative sparing of the MCP joints (Fig. 9–7). However, there may be extensive MCP joint and wrist involvement (Fig. 9–8). When the wrist is involved, as in any inflammatory arthritis, there is pancarpal involvement. In those patients with severe MCP and wrist involvement, one must use other criteria to distinguish the changes from those of rheumatoid arthritis (Fig. 9–9). There is usually extensive DIP involvement and/or evidence of bone proliferation. The distribution of psoriatic arthritis within the hand also differs from that of rheumatoid arthritis in that two or three rays may be involved, with sparing of the other rays (Fig. 9–10), whereas in rheumatoid arthritis all MCP's or all PIP joints are involved uniformly.

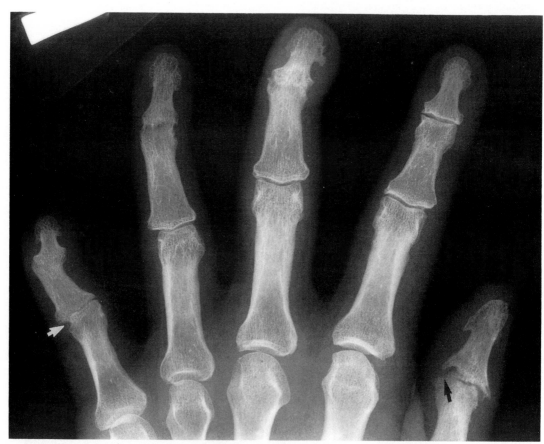

FIGURE 9–7. Involvement of IP joints with relative sparing of MCP joints. There is ankylosis of the 3rd, 4th, and 5th DIP joints and erosive changes (arrows) involving the IP joint of the thumb and the PIP joint of the 5th digit. (From Brower AC: The radiographic features of psoriatic arthritis. *In* Gerber L, Espinoza L (eds): Psoriatic Arthritis. Orlando, FL, Grune & Stratton, Inc, 1985, p 125.)

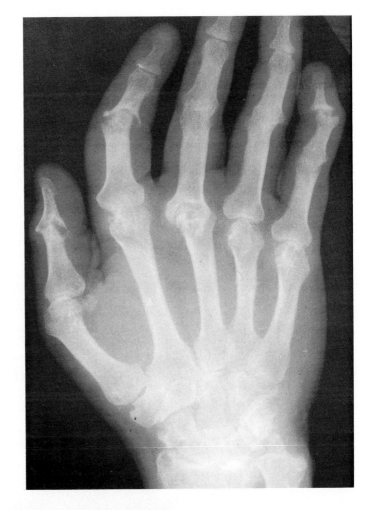

FIGURE 9–8. PA view of the hand in a patient with psoriatic arthritis. There is pancarpal involvement with erosive change. There is uniform MCP involvement with erosive change. However, note that the mineralization is normal. There is erosive change involving the DIP joint of the 5th digit and a pencil-in-cup erosion of the PIP joint of the 2nd digit. There is bone ankylosis of the 3rd, 4th, and 5th PIP joints.

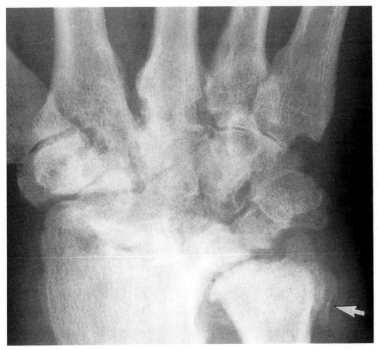

FIGURE 9–9. PA view of the wrist in a patient with psoriatic arthritis. There is pancarpal involvement with severe erosions of all the carpal bones. There is also evidence of bone ankylosis of the navicular to the capitate bone. However, evidence of bone production, best seen proximal to the ulnar styloid (arrow), distinguishes this psoriatic wrist from a wrist with rheumatoid arthritis. (From Brower AC: The radiographic features of psoriatic arthritis. In Gerber L, Espinoza L (eds): Psoriatic Arthritis. Orlando, FL, Grune & Stratton, Inc, 1985, p 125.)

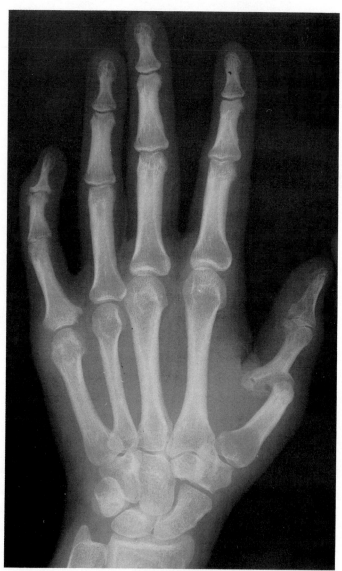

FIGURE 9–10. PA view of a hand with psoriatic arthritis. Note the involvement of the 1st and 5th rays, with sparing of the 2nd, 3rd, and 4th.

THE FEET

The radiographic changes described in the hand are also found in the feet. An entire digit may be swollen and resemble a sausage (Fig. 9–11). Although there may be early juxta-articular osteoporosis, generally the mineralization is maintained. Severe erosive changes with pencil pointing are observed. Extensive destruction of the IP joint of the great toe is more common in psoriatic arthritis than in any other arthritis (Fig. 9–12). Bone proliferation is identified as periostitis, new bone formation around erosions, and bone ankylosis of IP joints (Fig. 9–13). Bone proliferation around the distal phalanx of the great toe may produce an "ivory" phalanx (Fig. 9–14).

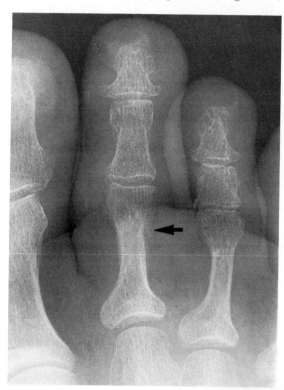

FIGURE 9–11. Soft tissue swelling of the entire 2nd digit. Note the fluffy periostitis (arrow) along the proximal phalanx. (From Brower AC: The radiographic features of psoriatic arthritis. *In* Gerber L, Espinoza L (eds): Psoriatic Arthritis. Orlando, Fl, Grune & Stratton, Inc, 1985, p 125.)

FIGURE 9–12. AP view of the forefoot in a patient with psoriatic arthritis. Note severe erosive changes of the DIP joints of the 2nd, 3rd, and 4th digits. There is ankylosis of the 2nd PIP joint. There is total destruction of the IP joint of the big toe with complete distortion of the distal end of the proximal phalanx. Note that mineralization is normal. (From Brower AC: The radiographic features of psoriatic arthritis. *In* Gerber L, Espinoza L (eds): Psoriatic Arthritis. Orlando, FL, Grune & Stratton, Inc, 1985, p 125.)

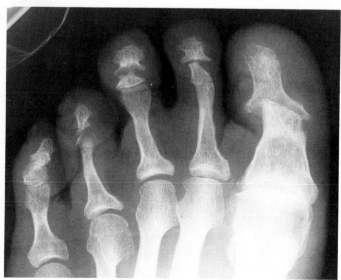

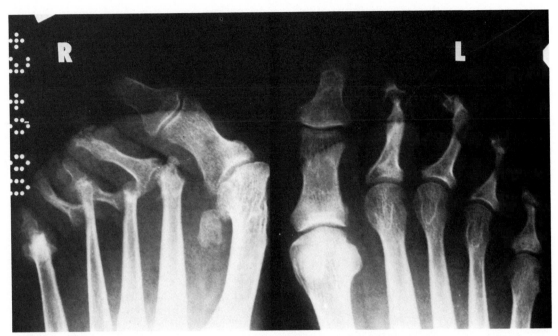

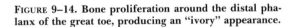

FIGURE 9–13. AP view of both forefeet in a patient with psoriatic arthritis. Note normal mineralization. There is pencil pointing of the distal metatarsals of the right foot, with subluxations and dislocations of the proximal phalanges. There is bone ankylosis of the PIP joint of the 2nd digit. In the left foot there is relative sparing of the MTP joints but severe involvement of the IP joints. Note the pencil pointing of the phalanges and the ankylosis of the PIP joints.

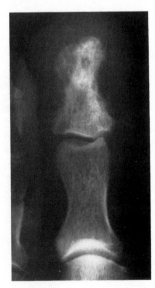

FIGURE 9–14. Bone proliferation around the distal phalanx of the great toe, producing an "ivory" appearance.

DIP and PIP involvement is common (Fig. 9–12). However, MTP involvement is more common than MCP involvement (Fig. 9–15). Again, two or three rays may be affected, with the other rays being spared.

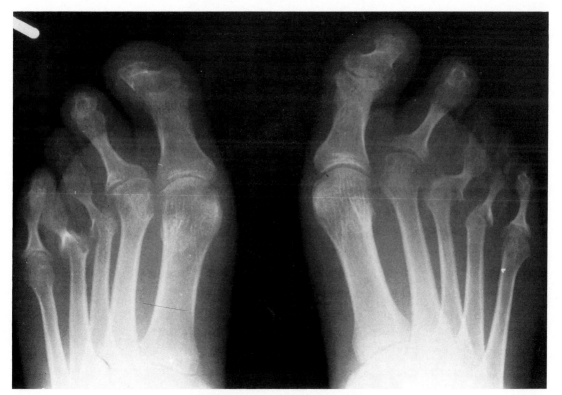

FIGURE 9–15. AP view of both forefeet in a patient with psoriatic arthritis. There is significant involvement of the MTP joints as well as ankylosis of the IP joints.

Radiographic changes are frequently seen on the posterior and inferior aspects of the calcaneus. Erosion and bone proliferation occur at the site of the Achilles tendon attachment posteriorly and superiorly (Fig. 9–16). Similar changes occur at the attachment of the plantar aponeurosis inferiorly, creating irregular and ill-defined spurs (Fig. 9–17). The spurs tend to point upward toward the calcaneus rather than downward along the course of the plantar aponeurosis as a normal heel spur points. Occasionally, the entire inferior aspect of the calcaneus may be involved.

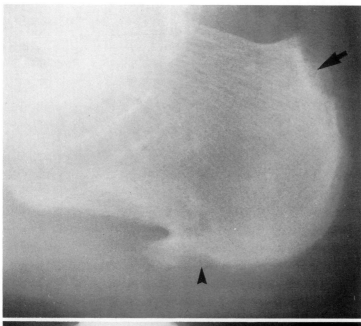

FIGURE 9–16. Erosion and bone production at the attachment of the Achilles tendon (arrow). There is also erosion of a calcaneal spur (arrowhead).

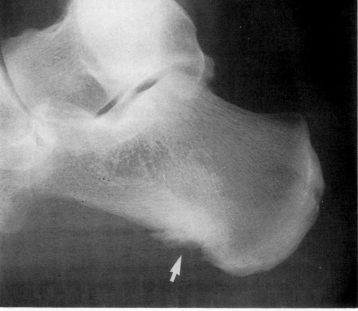

FIGURE 9–17. Erosion and bone proliferation at the attachment of the plantar aponeurosis (arrow). (From Brower AC: The radiographic features of psoriatic arthritis. *In* Gerber L, Espinoza L (eds): Psoriatic Arthritis. Orlando, FL, Grune & Stratton, Inc, 1985, p 125.)

OTHER APPENDICULAR SITES

The shoulder, elbow, knee, and ankle may be involved in psoriatic arthritis (Figs. 9–18 to 9–20). It is unusual for the hips to be affected. Bilateral but asymmetrical involvement is characteristic. Mineralization tends to be maintained. There is uniform loss of cartilage. Varying degrees of erosive changes and adjacent bone proliferation are characteristic. Bone proliferation at tendinous and ligamentous insertions is more frequently observed around the bigger joints. Common sites of proliferation are the femoral trochanters, the ischial tuberosities, the coracoclavicular ligament, the insertion of the rotator cuff, and the patellar tendons.

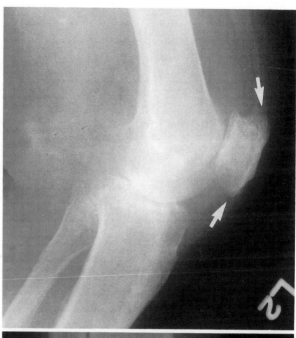

FIGURE 9–18. Lateral view of a knee in psoriatic arthritis. There is narrowing of the joint space and bone proliferation on anterior inferior, and superior surfaces of the patella (arrows).

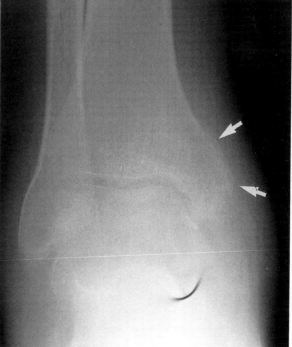

FIGURE 9–19. AP view of the ankle. Note soft tissue swelling. There is fluffy periosteal bone formation along the medial aspect of the distal tibia (arrow).

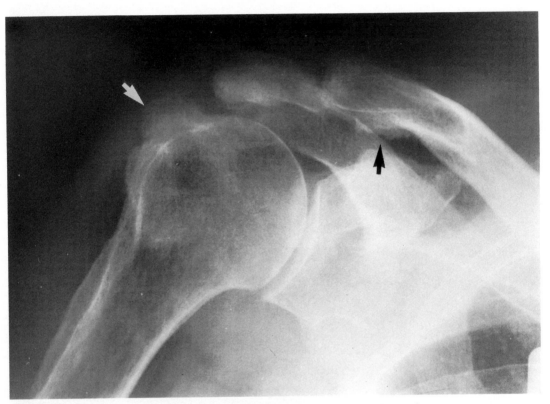

FIGURE 9–20. AP view of the shoulder in psoriatic arthritis. There is exuberant bone formation at tendon and ligamentous attachments (arrows). (From Brower AC: The radiographic features of psoriatic arthritis. *In* Gerber L, Espinoza L (eds): Psoriatic Arthritis. Orlando, FL, Grune & Stratton, Inc, 1985, p 125.)

THE SACROILIAC JOINTS

Thirty to 50 per cent of patients with psoriatic arthritis have involvement of their sacroiliac joints. Although the involvement may be bilateral and symmetrical, it is usually bilateral and asymmetrical, with one side being more involved than the other (Fig. 9–21). Initially, erosive changes are seen on the iliac side of the true synovial joint. As the erosions enlarge and involve the sacral side, proliferative bone repair is observed. The erosions and bone repair are more extensive than that seen with ankylosing spondylitis (Fig. 9–22). Bony ankylosis may occur across the joint, but much less frequently than is observed in ankylosing spondylitis.

Outside the true synovial joint, ossification of the ligaments between the sacrum and ilium may occur even without ankylosis of the synovial joint. Ossification of other tendinous attachments may be seen on the film of the pelvis: the iliac crest, the ischial tuberosities, and the femoral trochanters.

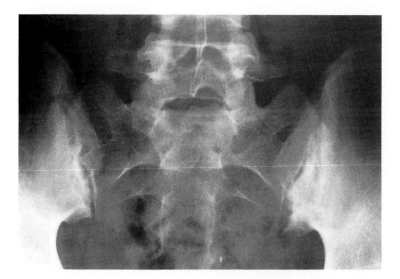

FIGURE 9–21. AP Ferguson view of the sacroiliac joints in psoriatic arthritis. There is bilateral but asymmetrical involvement consisting of erosions and reparative bone, predominantly on the iliac side. (From Brower AC: The radiographic features of psoriatic arthritis. *In* Gerber L, Espinoza L (eds): Psoriatic Arthritis. Orlando, FL, Grune & Stratton, Inc, 1985, p 125.)

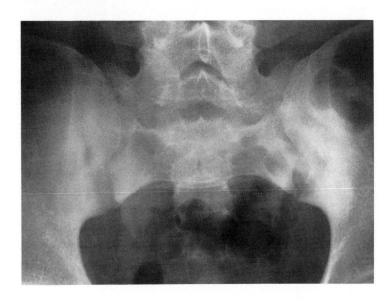

FIGURE 9–22. AP view of the sacroiliac joints in a patient with psoriatic arthritis. Large erosions and extensive bone repair are present.

THE SPINE

Spondylitis may occur with or without involvement of the sacroiliac joints. Involvement of the lumbar and thoracic spine is observed as paravertebral ossification. Large, bulky, bony outgrowths, unilateral or asymmetrical in their distribution, are characteristic and distinguish psoriasis from the succinct syndesmophyte of ankylosing spondylitis (Fig. 9–23). There is no squaring of the vertebral bodies and only occasional involvement of the apophyseal joints, two changes characteristic of ankylosing spondylitis.

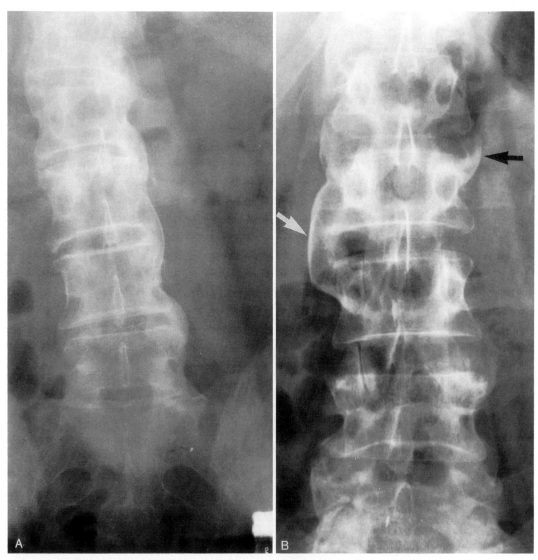

FIGURE 9–23. Psoriatic spondylitis. *A*, Asymmetrical, unilateral paravertebral ossifications. *B*, Large, bulky bone outgrowths joining underlying vertebral bodies. Note the asymmetrical distribution (arrows). (From Brower AC: The radiographic features of psoriatic arthritis. *In* Gerber L, Espinoza L (eds): Psoriatic Arthritis. Orlando, FL, Grune & Stratton, Inc, 1985, p 125.)

The cervical spine may be involved, with or without involvement of the rest of the spine. In the cervical spine the apophyseal joints are frequently affected, with narrowing, erosion, bone proliferation, and occasionally ankylosis (Fig. 9–24). There may be extensive bone proliferation along the anterior surface of the spine. Atlantoaxial subluxation, similar to that seen in rheumatoid arthritis, may also occur.

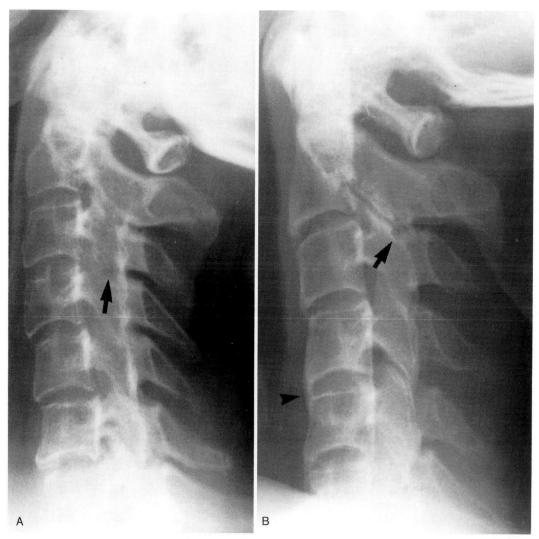

FIGURE 9–24. Cervical spine involvement in psoriatic arthritis. *A,* Apophyseal joint space narrowing, erosion (arrow), and ankylosis. *B,* Apophyseal joint space narrowing and erosion (arrow). There is also anterior paravertebral ossification present (arrowhead). (From Brower AC: The radiographic features of psoriatic arthritis. *In* Gerber L, Espinoza L (eds): Psoriatic Arthritis. Orlando, FL, Grune & Stratton, Inc, 1985, p 125.)

SUMMARY

Psoriatic arthritis presents specific radiographic changes in a specific distribution that allows the radiologist to make the diagnosis. It manifests a severe erosive element, as well as a bone productive element. The erosive changes help to distinguish it from ankylosing spondylitis and the bone productive changes, from rheumatoid arthritis.

SUGGESTED READINGS

Avila R, Pugh D, Slocumb CH, Winkelman RK: Psoriatic arthritis: A roentgenologic study. Radiology 75:691, 1960.

Fawcitt J: Bone and joint changes associated with psoriasis. Br J Radiol 23:440, 1950.

Harvie JN, Lester RS, Little AH: Sacroiliitis in severe psoriasis. AJR 127:579, 1976.

Jajic I: Radiological changes in the sacroiliac joints and spine of patients with psoriatic arthritis and psoriasis. Ann Rheum Dis 27:1, 1968.

Killebrew K, Gold RH, Sholkoff SD: Psoriatic spondylitis. Radiology 108:9, 1973.

Meaney TF, Hays RA: Roentgen manifestations of psoriatic arthritis. Radiology 68:403, 1957.

Peterson CC Jr, Silbiger ML: Reiter's syndrome and psoriatic arthritis: Their roentgen spectra and some interesting similarities. AJR 101:860, 1967.

Resnick D, Broderick RW: Bony proliferation of terminal phalanges in psoriasis: The "ivory" phalanx. J Can Assoc Radiol 28:187, 1977.

Resnick D, Niwayama G: On the nature and significance of bony proliferation in "rheumatoid variant" disorders. AJR 129:275, 1977.

Resnick D, Niwayama G: Psoriatic arthritis. In Resnick D, Niwayama G (eds.): Diagnosis of Bone and Joint Disorders. Vol. 2. Philadelphia, W. B. Saunders Company, 1981, p 1103.

Sherman MS: Psoriatic arthritis. Observations on the clinical, roentgenographic, and pathological changes. J Bone Joint Surg 34A:831, 1952.

Wright V: Psoriatic arthritis. A comparative radiographic study of rheumatoid arthritis and arthritis associated with psoriasis. Ann Rheum Dis 20:123, 1961.

chapter 10

REITER'S
DISEASE

The arthritis of Reiter's syndrome is usually associated with conjunctivitis and urethritis. It is a disease predominantly of males between 15 and 35 years of age and is transmitted through either epidemic dysentery or sexual intercourse. In today's military population the arthritis may be present without documentation of the other clinical manifestations. In such cases, radiographic examination may provide the appropriate diagnosis. The classic radiographic features are as follows:

1. **Fusiform soft tissue swelling**

2. **Early juxta-articular osteoporosis; re-establishment of normal mineralization**

3. **Uniform joint space loss**

4. **Bone proliferation**

5. **Ill-defined erosions**

6. **Bilateral asymmetrical distribution**

7. **Distribution primarily in feet, ankles, knees, and sacroiliac joints; hands, hips, and spine less frequently involved**

Although the specific radiographic changes are identical to those of psoriatic arthritis, Reiter's arthritis has a characteristic but different distribution, thus allowing for accurate differential diagnosis.

THE FEET

The small articulations of the foot and the calcaneus are the most frequently involved joints in the arthritis of Reiter's disease. The arthritis is initially seen involving one joint only (Fig. 10–1). This monarticular involvement could lead to a misdiagnosis of septic arthritis; therefore, the observation of the aggressiveness of the changes plays an important role in correct interpretation. There may be swelling of the entire digit, giving it an appearance of a "sausage" or "cocktail hotdog." Early in the disease juxta-articular osteoporosis is present and persists for a longer period of time than it does in psoriasis. Eventually normal mineralization returns. Early, a periostitis may be observed along the shafts of the phalanges (Fig. 10–2). Later, uniform joint space loss and marginal erosions with adjacent bone proliferation occur (Fig. 10–3). These changes are indistinguishable from the changes of psoriatic arthritis in the toes. Ankylosis of the joints does not occur as frequently as it does in psoriatic arthritis. Reiter's arthritis also seems to prefer the MTP joints (Fig. 10–4) and 1st IP joint over the DIP and PIP joints seen classically in psoriatic arthritis.

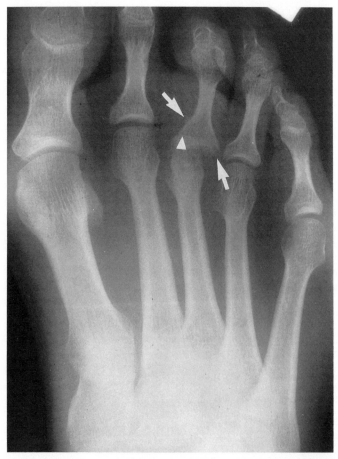

FIGURE 10–1. AP view of the forefoot in Reiter's arthritis. There is monarticular involvement of the 3rd MTP joint. There is superimposition of the proximal end of the proximal phalanx and the distal end of the metatarsal head, indicative of subluxation. There is new bone formation around the proximal phalanx (arrows). There is erosive change involving the juxta-articular areas of the metatarsal head. The white cortical line of the articular surface of the 3rd metatarsal head (arrowhead) is intact, indicating a process less aggressive than septic arthritis.

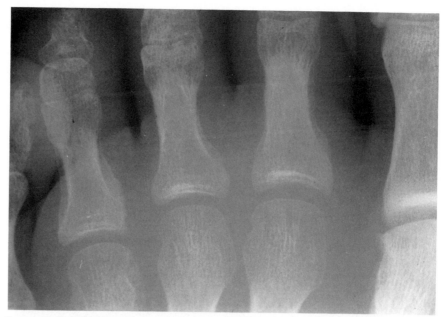

FIGURE 10–2. MTP joints in Reiter's disease. There is juxta-articular osteoporosis present. Periostitis is present along the shafts of the 2nd, 3rd, and 4th proximal phalanges.

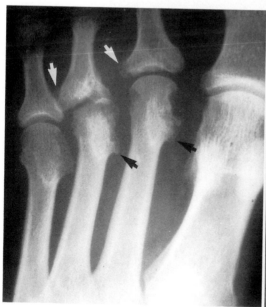

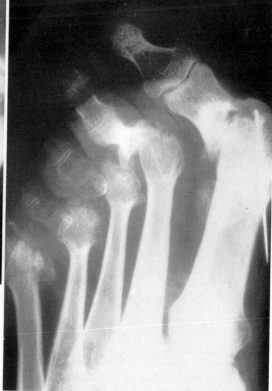

FIGURE 10–3. AP view of the 1st through 4th toes in a patient with Reiter's arthritis. The 2nd and 3rd MTP joints are involved with erosive disease and adjacent bone proliferation (arrows).

FIGURE 10–4. An AP view of the foot in Reiter's disease. There is dramatic involvement of all of the MTP joints with juxta-articular osteoporosis, subluxations, erosive disease, and adjacent bone proliferation. The IP joints are relatively spared.

The calcaneus is involved in more than 50 per cent of patients with Reiter's disease. Often it may be the only bone ever involved and hence the name "lover's heel." As in psoriatic arthritis, there is erosion and bone production at the attachment of the Achilles tendon and the plantar aponeurosis. Ill-defined spurs may develop at the aponeurotic attachment more frequently than at the Achilles tendon attachment (Fig. 10–5). They will tend to point upward toward the calcaneus (Fig. 10–6).

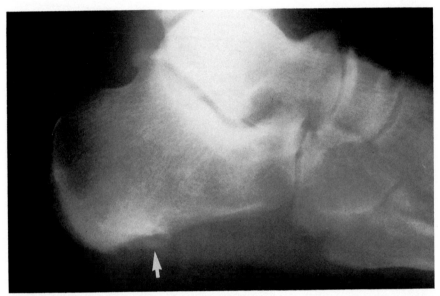

FIGURE 10–5. Lateral view of the calcaneus in Reiter's disease. There is erosive change at the attachment of the plantar aponeurosis. There is adjacent proliferative bone production (arrow).

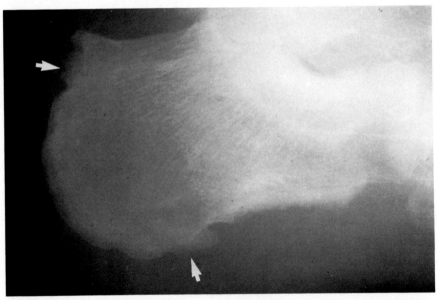

FIGURE 10–6. Lateral view of the calcaneus in a patient with long-standing Reiter's arthritis. There are erosive changes at both the attachment of the Achilles tendon and the plantar aponeurosis. There is associated bone production (arrows). The calcaneal spur is pointing slightly toward the calcaneus.

THE ANKLES

One or both ankles may be involved in 30 to 50 per cent of the patients with Reiter's disease (Fig. 10–7). There are usually soft tissue swelling and a fluffy periostitis involving the distal ends of the fibula and tibia. Uniform joint space loss may occur. Erosive disease is a less frequent manifestation.

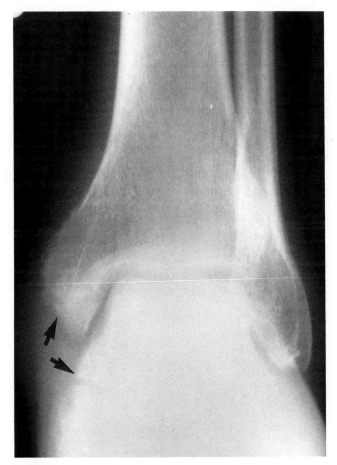

FIGURE 10–7. AP view of the ankle involved with Reiter's arthritis. There is soft tissue swelling around the ankle. There is proliferative periostitis over the medial malleolus and talus (arrows).

THE KNEES

Forty per cent of the patients with Reiter's disease have involvement of one or both knees. The most common finding is the presence of a joint effusion. Juxta-articular osteoporosis may be observed, although eventually this is replaced with normal mineralization. Bone production observed as a periostitis or ossification of ligamentous and tendinous attachments is more common than erosive disease.

OTHER APPENDICULAR SITES

Whereas involvement of the joints of the lower extremities is common, involvement of the hip is relatively rare. Involvement of one or more joints in the upper extremity usually occurs before involvement of the hip. The most common area of involvement in the upper extremity is the hand. This is often limited to one digit (Fig. 10–8), although certainly several digits and/or the wrist may be involved (Fig. 10–9). Again the specific radiographic changes are identical to those seen in psoriatic arthritis with erosive disease and evidence of new bone formation. There is a tendency toward persistent juxta-articular osteoporosis. Ankylosis of the IP joints is less frequent. The PIP joints are more frequently involved than the DIP's or MCP's.

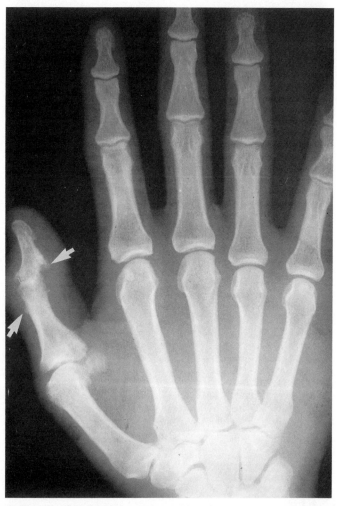

FIGURE 10–8. PA view of the hand in a patient with Reiter's arthritis. The only abnormality is the involvement of the IP joint and MCP joint of the thumb. There is soft tissue swelling around the IP joint with uniform loss of the joint space, erosive changes, and associated bone productive changes (arrow). There is joint space loss in the 1st MCP joint. There are bone productive changes seen around the sesamoid bone.

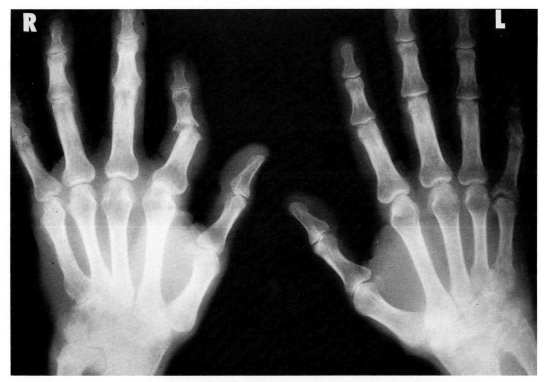

FIGURE 10–9. PA view of the hands in a patient with Reiter's arthritis. There is pancarpal involvement bilaterally. The PIP joints are involved with extensive changes at the 2nd PIP joint on the right and the 5th PIP joint on the left. The MCP's are involved to a lesser extent, with the most dramatic changes being in the left 5th MCP joint.

THE SACROILIAC JOINTS

Early in the course of the disease the sacroiliac joint is affected in 5 to 10 per cent of patients; however, several years into the course of the disease, 40 to 60 per cent have sacroiliac involvement. Although the involvement may be bilateral and symmetrical, it is usually bilateral and asymmetrical, with one side more extensively involved than the other (Fig. 10–10). Because of this asymmetrical involvement, radiographically it may appear as a unilateral involvement (Fig. 10–11). It then becomes important to distinguish Reiter's disease from septic arthritis of the sacroiliac joint. Bone scintigraphy aids immensely in establishing the correct diagnosis; in Reiter's disease, even though the radiographic changes may be unilateral, both sacroiliac joints show increased uptake on the scan. As with psoriatic arthritis, erosive changes are first seen on the iliac side of the true synovial joint. As the erosions enlarge and involve the sacral side, proliferative bone repair is observed. Both may become quite extensive (Fig. 10–10). Ankylosis of the sacroiliac joint occurs less frequently than in psoriatic arthritis.

In addition to the changes in the sacroiliac joints, similar changes may occur at the pubic symphysis. Ossification of tendinous attachments may also be observed.

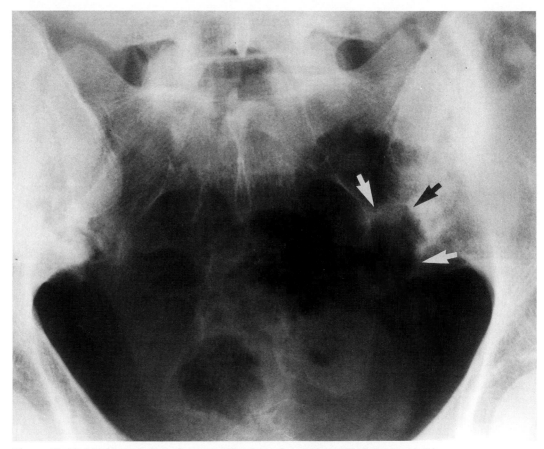

FIGURE 10–10. AP Ferguson view of the sacroiliac joints in a patient with Reiter's arthritis. There is bilateral asymmetrical involvement. Bone sclerosis is the prominent feature on the right side. A large erosion is seen in the inferior aspect of the left SI joint (arrows). (From Brower AC: Disorders of the sacroiliac joint. Radiolog 1(20):3, 1978.)

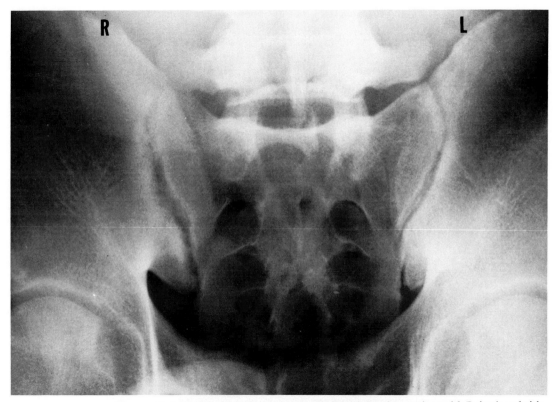

FIGURE 10–11. AP Ferguson view of the sacroiliac joints in a patient with Reiter's arthritis. The left sacroiliac joint is within normal limits. The right sacroiliac joint shows early changes of small erosions and adjacent sclerosis on the iliac side.

THE SPINE

Involvement of the spine in Reiter's disease is relatively rare and certainly less frequent than in psoriatic arthritis. Early spinal involvement occurs as paravertebral ossification somewhere around the lower three thoracic or upper three lumbar vertebral bodies (Fig. 10–12). In this location, if such ossification progresses, one observes large bulky bone bridges between adjacent vertebral bodies. As in psoriasis, their distribution will be unilateral or asymmetrical. As in psoriasis, there will be no squaring of the vertebral bodies and only occasional involvement of the apophyseal joints. In contrast to psoriasis, involvement of the cervical spine is extremely rare.

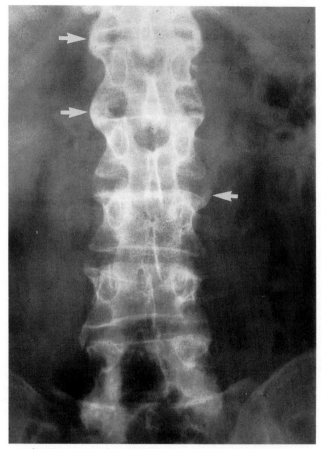

FIGURE 10–12. AP view of the lumbar spine in a patient with Reiter's arthritis. There is paravertebral ossification at the T12-L1, L1-L2, and L2-L3 disc spaces (arrows).

SUMMARY

The specific radiographic changes of Reiter's arthritis are indistinguishable from those of psoriatic arthritis. There is a tendency toward more juxta-articular osteoporosis and less ankylosis than in psoriatic arthritis. However, its characteristic lower extremity distribution is the most useful manifestation in distinguishing it from psoriatic arthritis.

SUGGESTED READINGS

Mason RM, Murray RS, Oates JK, Young AC: A comparative radiological study of Reiter's disease, rheumatoid arthritis, and ankylosing spondylitis. J Bone Joint Surg 41B:137, 1959.

Murray RS, Oates JK, Young AC: Radiologic changes in Reiter's syndrome and arthritis associated with urethritis. J Fac Radiologists 9:37, 1958.

Peterson CC Jr, Silbiger ML: Reiter's syndrome and psoriatic arthritis. Their roentgen spectra and some interesting similarities. AJR 101:860, 1967.

Resnick D, Niwayama G: Reiter's syndrome. In Resnick D, Niwayama G (eds.): Diagnosis of Bone and Joint Disorders. Vol. 2. Philadelphia, W. B. Saunders Company, 1981, p 1130.

Reynolds DF, Csonka GW: Radiological aspects of Reiter's syndrome ("venereal" arthritis). J Fac Radiologists 9:44, 1958.

Sholkoff SD, Glickman MG, Steinback HL: Roentgenology of Reiter's syndrome. Radiology 97:497, 1970.

Sundaram M, Patton JT: Paravertebral ossification in psoriasis and Reiter's disease. Br J Radiol 48:628, 1975.

Weldon WV, Scalettar R: Roentgen changes in Reiter's syndrome. AJR 86:344, 1961.

chapter 11

ANKYLOSING SPONDYLITIS

Ankylosing spondylitis is the chronic inflammatory disease that primarily affects the axial skeleton and only secondarily the appendicular skeleton. It is seen predominantly in men between the ages of 15 and 35 years. Of all the inflammatory arthropathies, it is the least erosive and the most ossifying. Ankylosis of a joint is the predominant characteristic. The common radiographic findings are as follows:

1. Normal mineralization before ankylosis; generalized osteoporosis after ankylosis

2. Subchondral bone formation present before ankylosis

3. Erosions—small, localized, and not a prominent part of the picture

4. Absence of subluxations

5. Absence of cysts

6. Ankylosis

7. Bilateral symmetrical distribution

8. Distribution in sacroiliac joints and the spine, ascending from the lumbar to the cervical; then hips, shoulders, knees, hands, and feet in decreasing order of frequency

The axial distribution and the predominant ankylosing features make the radiographic diagnosis relatively easy.

THE SACROILIAC JOINTS

Although clinically ankylosing spondylitis is first suspected because of involvement of the costovertebral junction, radiographically the first involvement is seen in the sacroiliac joints. They are involved in a bilateral and symmetrical fashion (Fig. 11–1). Small succinct erosions are seen first on the iliac side and then on the sacral side, giving the joint margin the appearance of the perforated edge of a postage stamp (Fig. 11–2). The erosions are surrounded by a small amount of bone repair. The erosions and sclerosis never become as extensive as those seen in the other spondyloarthropathies. The synovial aspect of the joint will ankylose relatively early. It is common for the entire sacroiliac joint, not only the true synovial aspect but also the ligamentous aspect, to ankylose. The ossification of the ligaments in the posterior superior portion of the sacroiliac joint is seen radiographically as a "star" (Fig. 11–3).

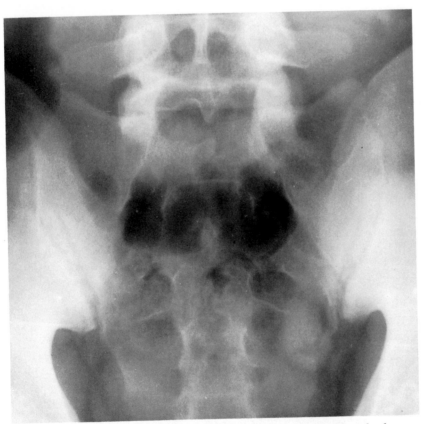

FIGURE 11–1. AP Ferguson view of the sacroiliac joints in a patient with early changes of ankylosing spondylitis. There is bilateral and symmetrical involvement. The erosions are succinct. There is minimal sclerosis. (From Brower AC: Disorders of the sacroiliac joint. Radiology 1(20):3, 1978.)

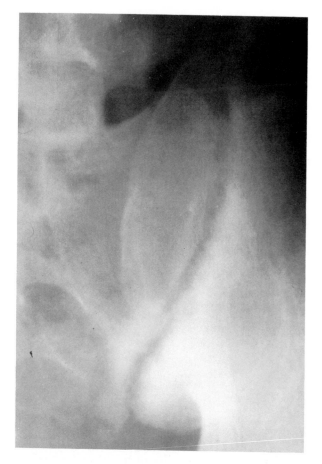

FIGURE 11–2. AP view of the sacroiliac joint in early ankylosing spondylitis. The erosions are small, giving the joint edge the appearance of the perforated edge of a postage stamp. A small amount of bone repair is present.

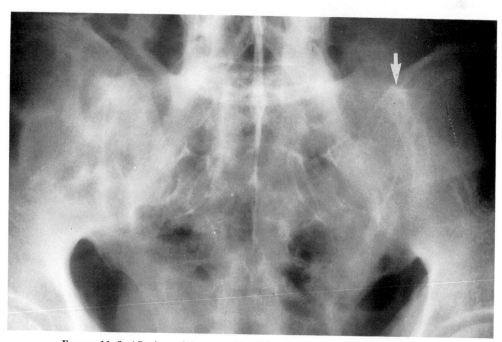

FIGURE 11–3. AP view of the sacroiliac joints in a patient with long-standing ankylosing spondylitis. Both SI joints are completely ankylosed. A "star" (arrow) represents the ossification of the ligaments in the posterior superior portion of the joint.

Other changes in the pelvis may be seen concurrent with the changes in the sacroiliac joints. There may be ossification of the ligamentous attachments to the iliac crest and ischial tuberosities, giving a "whiskered" appearance (Fig. 11–15). The pubic symphysis may be involved, with small succinct erosions and reparative response adjacent to the erosions, followed by total ankylosis (Fig. 11–4). The pubic symphysis is involved in 23 per cent of patients.

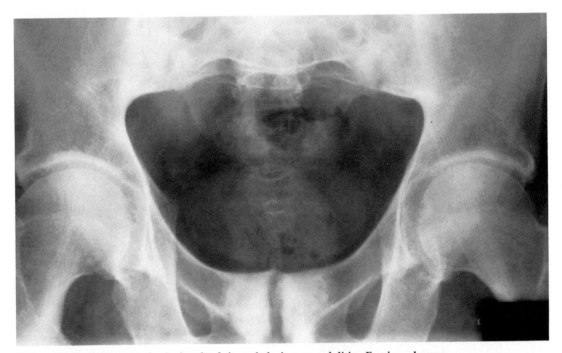

FIGURE 11–4. Pubic symphysis involved in ankylosing spondylitis. Erosive changes producing apparent widening and adjacent reparative response.

THE SPINE

Initial involvement of the spine may be seen in the T12-L1 area. However, usually spine involvement is identified by the radiologist in the lumbar area. It is then seen to progress upward through the thoracic spine to the cervical spine. Initially there is erosion of the corner of the vertebral body with secondary reactive sclerosis. This gives a squared appearance to the vertebral body, and the reactive sclerosis is identified as the ivory corner (Fig. 11–5). As the spine becomes immobilized, this reactive sclerosis disappears and one may identify nothing more than a squared vertebral body.

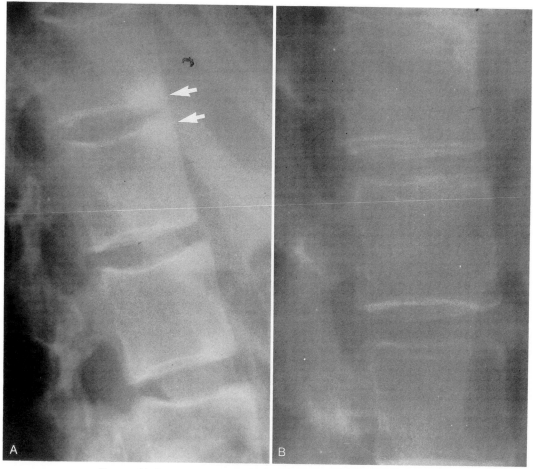

FIGURE 11–5. *A*, Erosion of the corner of the vertebral bodies and resultant reactive sclerosis give a squared appearance to the vertebral bodies and ivory corners (arrows). *B*, Reactive sclerosis has disappeared owing to immobility. Squaring of the vertebral bodies is the only abnormality seen.

Ossification first takes place in the outer portion of the anulus fibrosus or in Sharpey's fibers. At first this ossification may not be visible radiographically, but lack of motion on flexion and extension films will indicate its presence (Fig. 11–6). This ossification will extend from Sharpey's fibers into the deep layers of the longitudinal ligaments. This ossification is called a syndesmophyte and ossifies one vertebral body to the adjacent vertebral body in a succinct fashion (Fig. 11–7). The syndesmophytes ascend the lumbar spine in a symmetrical fashion to eventually involve the thoracic spine and the cervical spine (Fig. 11–8). The disc spaces are generally preserved. Once ankylosis has taken place disc calcification may develop (Fig. 11–9).

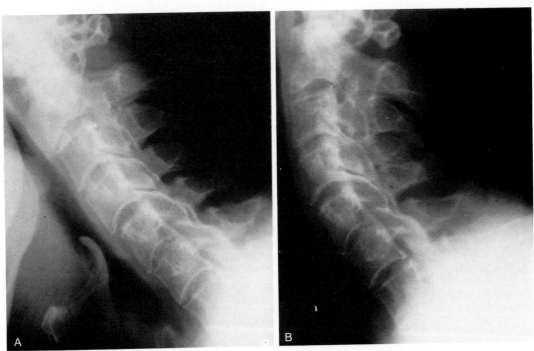

FIGURE 11–6. Lateral views of the cervical spine in ankylosing spondylitis. *A*, Flexion and (*B*) extension views. Despite the lack of visible ossification of the anulus fibrosus and/or anterior longitudinal ligament, there is no demonstrable motion between C5 and C6 or C6 and C7.

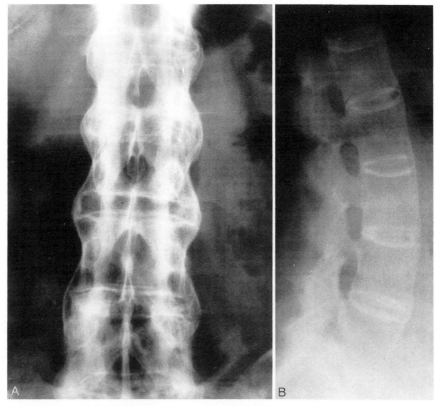

FIGURE 11–7. *A*, AP and (*B*) lateral views of lumbar vertebral bodies showing succinct syndesmophytes of ankylosing spondylitis.

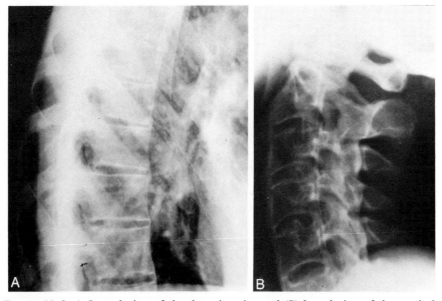

FIGURE 11–8. *A*, Lateral view of the thoracic spine and (*B*) lateral view of the cervical spine showing succinct ossification of the anulus fibrosus and deep layers of the anterior longitudinal ligament in ankylosing spondylitis.

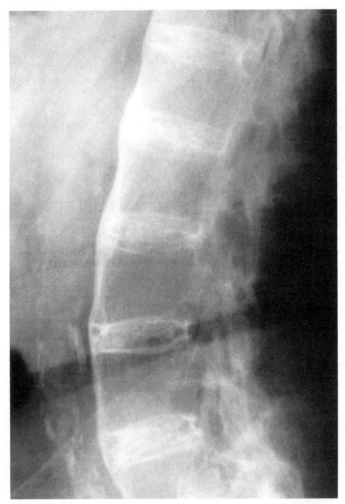

FIGURE 11–9. Lateral view of the lumbar spine in long-standing ankylosing spondylitis. Note the succinct syndesmophyte formation. There is calcification of all discs.

The apophyseal joints may or may not be involved with erosive change and adjacent bone repair followed by ankylosis (Fig. 11–10). Ossification of all ligaments, including those between the spinous processes, may be present. The resulting appearance is that of a bamboo spine (Fig. 11–11).

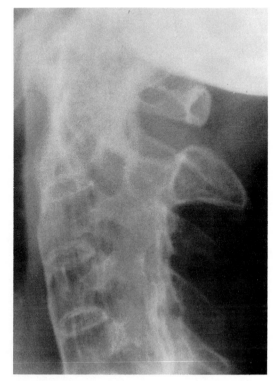

FIGURE 11–10. Lateral view of the cervical spine showing syndesmophytes, osteoporosis, and ankylosis of the apophyseal joints.

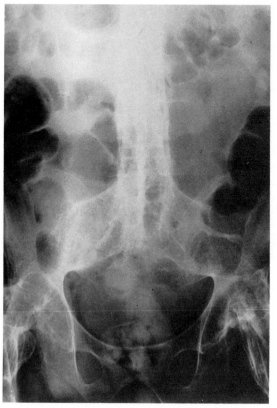

FIGURE 11–11. AP view of the lumbar spine and pelvis in a patient with long-standing ankylosing spondylitis. This is a classic bamboo spine. There is syndesmophyte formation and ossification of the ligaments between the spinous processes. There is ankylosis of the SI joints, the pubic symphysis, and both hips.

In the cervical spine erosion of the odontoid process may occur. Atlanto-axial subluxation may also be demonstrated on flexed views taken in the lateral projection. While these two findings are characteristic of rheumatoid arthritis, involvement of the rest of the spine with ankylosis should prevent erroneous diagnosis. Intubation of a patient with ankylosing spondylitis involving the cervical spine can result in a disastrous fracture if the intubater is unaware of the presence of the disease process (Fig. 11–12).

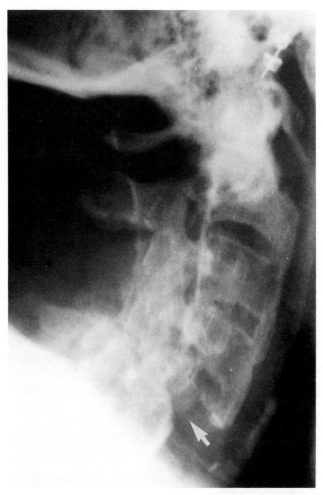

FIGURE 11–12. Lateral view of the cervical spine in a patient with ankylosing spondylitis. Note the fracture at C4-C5 (arrow) incurred during intubation.

A common misdiagnosed complication of the bamboo spine is the pseudarthrosis that may develop in the lower thoracic–upper lumbar spine area. This develops around an area of true fracture or an area of skipped ossification (Fig. 11–13). It becomes the single point of motion in the entire spine and therefore undergoes disc degeneration and disintegration, erosion, and eburnation. The changes can resemble those of severe degenerated disc, a septic discitis and osteomyelitis, or a neuropathic spine (Fig. 11–14). The etiology of these radiographic changes must be understood so that the correct diagnosis can be made.

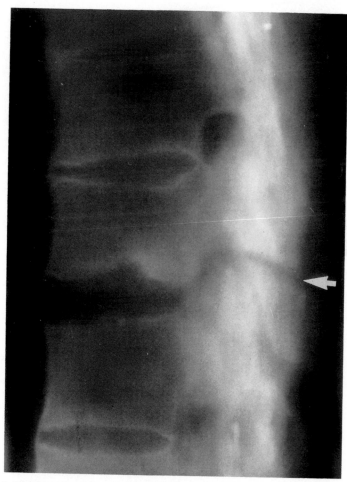

FIGURE 11–13. Tomographic cut taken in the lateral plane through the lower thoracic–upper lumbar spine area. There is ankylosis of the entire spine, except at T12-L1 (arrow). Here, there is distraction (widening) of the disc space and fracture through the posterior elements. (Courtesy of Dr. C. S. Resnik, University of Maryland.)

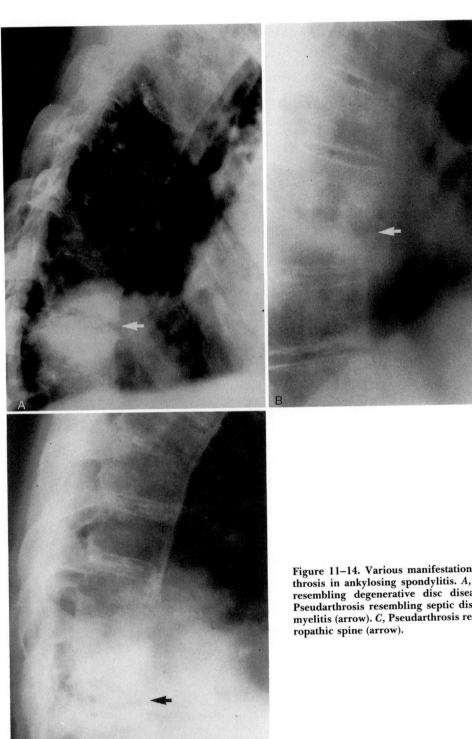

Figure 11–14. Various manifestations of a pseudarthrosis in ankylosing spondylitis. *A*, Pseudarthrosis resembling degenerative disc disease (arrow). *B*, Pseudarthrosis resembling septic discitis and osteomyelitis (arrow). *C*, Pseudarthrosis resembling a neuropathic spine (arrow).

THE HIP

After the axial skeleton, the most common joint to be involved is the hip joint. Two different types of involvement are described: the non-destructive and the destructive. The non-destructive is the more common type of involvement. It is seen in the younger patient. There is a bilateral symmetrical involvement of both hips, with ankylosis a prominent part of the picture. There may be no loss of joint space, or there may be uniform loss of joint space with axial migration of the femoral head within the acetabulum. Very superficial erosions may be present, but basically the normal round contour of the femoral head is not distorted. Before true ankylosis takes place, normal mineralization will be present and a collar of osteophytes will be seen at the junction of the head and neck (Fig. 11–15). Once ankylosis has taken place the surrounding bone becomes osteoporotic, and this cuff of osteophytes disappears (Fig. 11–16).

The less common type of involvement of the hip tends to be a unilateral involvement. The progression of change is much slower. There is considerable destruction of the femoral head, with marked irregularity of the contour developing before progression to ankylosis.

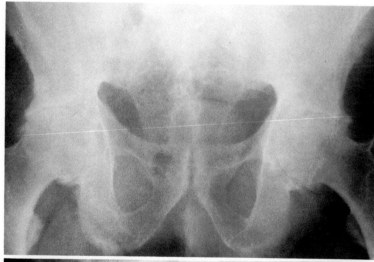

FIGURE 11–15. AP view of the pelvis in a patient with ankylosing spondylitis. Normal mineralization is present. Both hips demonstrate uniform loss of cartilage with axial migration. A cuff of osteophytes is present at the junction of the head and neck as well as on the inferior and superior aspects of the acetabulum. There is ankylosis of the sacroiliac joints. There is ossification of the ligamentous attachments to the ischial tuberosities, giving a "whiskered" appearance.

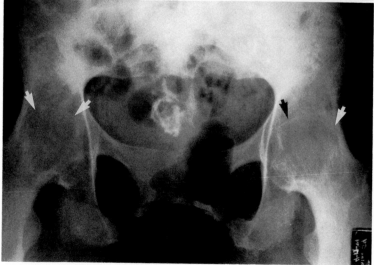

FIGURE 11–16. AP view of the pelvis in a patient with long-standing ankylosing spondylitis. There is generalized osteoporosis. There is ankylosis of the SI joints, the pubic symphysis, and both hips. Note that the normal round contour of the femoral head is seen through the ankylosis (arrows).

THE SHOULDER

After the hip, the shoulder is the next most commonly involved joint. Again, there are two types of involvement, the non-destructive and the destructive. The non-destructive type shows a normally shaped humeral head ankylosed to the glenoid and extensive ossification of the coracoclavicular ligament (Fig. 11–17). The less common destructive type shows a large hatchet-shaped erosion of the humeral head. Eventually ankylosis takes place, but not until the destruction has occurred.

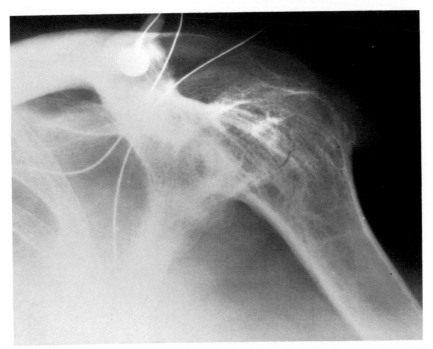

FIGURE 11–17. AP view of the shoulder in long-standing ankylosing spondylitis. The humeral head is ankylosed to the glenoid. There is extensive ossification of the coracoclavicular ligament.

OTHER JOINTS

The acromioclavicular, sternoclavicular, and sternomanubrial joints are commonly affected joints. The knee is affected in 30 per cent of patients with long-standing disease (Fig. 11–18). The elbow, hands, and feet are affected in approximately 10 per cent of patients with long-standing disease (Fig. 11–19). In all of these areas, if erosive disease exists, the erosions are relatively superficial with minimal reparative bone response. The hallmark is always intra-articular ankylosis in a relatively short period of time.

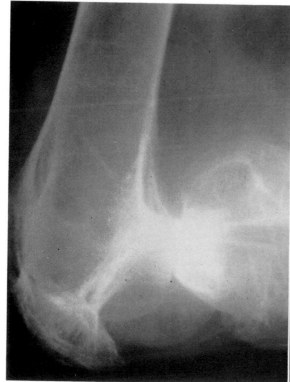

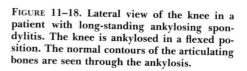

FIGURE 11–18. Lateral view of the knee in a patient with long-standing ankylosing spondylitis. The knee is ankylosed in a flexed position. The normal contours of the articulating bones are seen through the ankylosis.

FIGURE 11–19. Lateral view of the hand in a patient with ankylosing spondylitis, showing ankylosis of all visible joints.

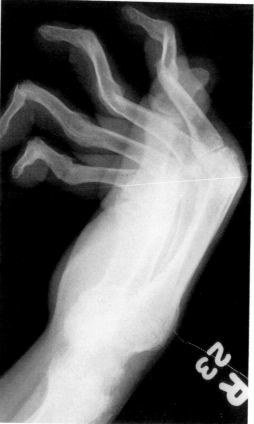

SUMMARY

The radiographic diagnosis of ankylosing spondylitis should not be a problem. Its predominance in the axial skeleton and its intra-articular ankylosis in a short period of time are classic and pathognomonic.

SUGGESTED READINGS

Berens DL: Roentgen features of ankylosing spondylitis. Clin Orthop 71:20, 1971.

Cawley MID, Chalmers IM, Kellgren JH, Ball J: Destructive lesions of vertebral bodies in ankylosing spondylitis. Ann Rheum Dis 31:345, 1972.

Dihlmann W: Current radiodiagnostic concept of ankylosing spondylitis. Skeletal Radiol 4:179–188, 1979.

Dwosh IL, Resnick D, Becker MA: Hip involvement in ankylosing spondylitis. Arthritis Rheum 19:683, 1976.

Edeiken J, Depalma A, Hodes PJ: Ankylosing spondylitis. Clin Orthop 34:62, 1984.

Forestier F: The importance of sacroiliac changes in early diagnosis of ankylosing spondyloarthritis. Radiology 33:389, 1939.

Martel W: Diagnostic radiology in the rheumatic diseases. In Kelley WN, Harris ED, Ruddy S, et al. (eds.): Textbook of Rheumatology. Philadelphia, W. B. Saunders Company, 1981.

McEwen C, Ditata D, Longg C, et al.: Ankylosing spondylitis and the spondylitis accompanying ulcerative colitis, regional enteritis, psoriasis and Reiter's disease. A comparative study. Arthritis Rheum 14:291, 1971.

Resnick D: Patterns of peripheral joint disease in ankylosing spondylitis. Radiology 110:523, 1974.

Resnick D, Niwayama G: Ankylosing spondylitis. In Resnick D, Niwayama G (eds.): Diagnosis of Bone and Joint Disorders. Vol. 2. Philadelphia, W. B. Saunders Company, 1981.

Rivelis M, Freiberger RH: Vertebral destruction at unfused segments in late ankylosing spondylitis. Radiology 93:251, 1969.

chapter 12

OSTEOARTHRITIS

Osteoarthritis is the most common arthropathy seen today. While many arthropathies lead to secondary osteoarthritic changes, this chapter deals with primary osteoarthritis and osteoarthritis secondary to alteration of normal mechanics across a weight-bearing joint. The radiographic hallmarks of osteoarthritis are as follows:

1. **Normal mineralization**

2. **Non-uniform loss of joint space**

3. **Absence of erosions**

4. **Subchondral new bone formation**

5. **Osteophyte formation**

6. **Cysts**

7. **Subluxations**

8. **Unilateral and/or bilateral asymmetrical distribution**

9. **Distribution in hands, feet, knees, hips; sparing of shoulders and elbows**

Except for the type of joint space loss, all of the above features may also be seen in osteoarthritis developing secondary to an underlying cartilage problem. In secondary osteoarthritis the joint space loss is uniform; in primary or mechanical osteoarthritis the joint space loss is non-uniform.

THE HAND

Primary osteoarthritis in the hand involves the DIP and PIP joints with relative sparing of the MCP joints (Fig. 12–1). The soft tissue swelling around the DIP joint associated with osteophyte formation is called a Heberdon node (Fig. 12–2); that around the PIP joint is called a Bouchard node. There is non-uniform loss of the joint space with subchondral sclerosis and osteophyte development in the area of greatest loss of cartilage. The osteophyte must not be confused with either the new bone formation of psoriasis or the saucerized flared edge of the bone caused by erosion of psoriasis. An osteophyte is an extension of a normal articular surface. In the IP joints the osteophyte extends laterally or medially and proximally toward the body (Fig. 12–3). Erosion and ankylosis, manifestations of inflammatory disease, are not present. Cyst formation is relatively rare in the digits.

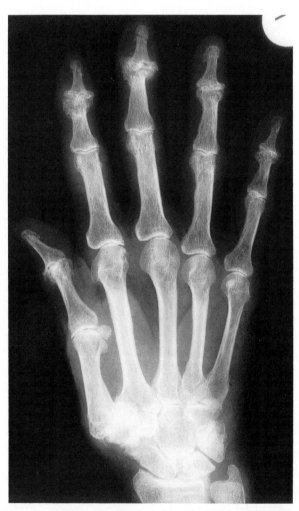

FIGURE 12–1. PA view of the hand in osteoarthritis. The DIP joints are primarily involved with cartilage loss, osteophyte formation, and subchondral sclerosis. The wrist shows involvement of the base of the 1st metacarpal as it articulates with the greater multangular and the greater multangular as it articulates with the navicular. Again there are subchondral sclerosis and osteophyte formation. (From Brower AC: The radiologic approach to arthritis. Med Clin North Am 68:1593, 1984.)

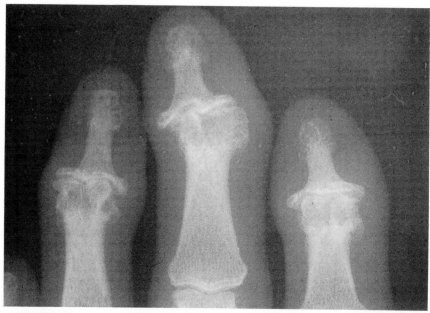

FIGURE 12–2. DIP joints in osteoarthritis. The soft tissue swelling associated with the osteophyte formation is called a Heberdon node.

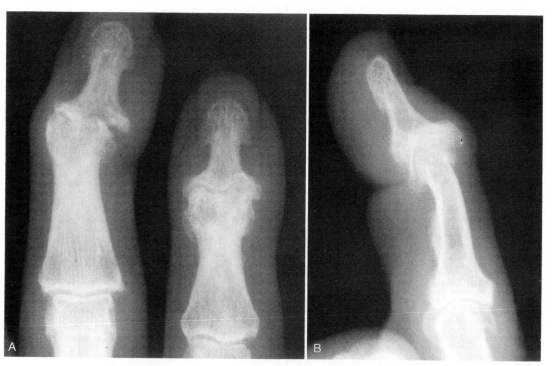

FIGURE 12–3. *A*, PA view of DIP joints showing non-uniform loss of joint space, subchondral sclerosis, and osteophyte formation extending laterally and medially. *B*, Lateral view of IP joints showing osteophytes extending proximally toward the body.

Primary osteoarthritis of the wrist involves only two joints: that between the base of the 1st metacarpal and the greater multangular and that between the greater multangular and the navicular (Fig. 12–4). There may be radial subluxation of the base of the 1st metacarpal in relationship to the greater multangular (Fig. 12–5). Large osteophyte formation is seen between the base of the 1st and 2nd metacarpals. Eburnation and cyst formation are present. Osteoarthritic changes involving any other joint in the wrist must be considered secondary to another arthropathy, e.g., calcium pyrophosphate dihydrate crystal deposition disease.

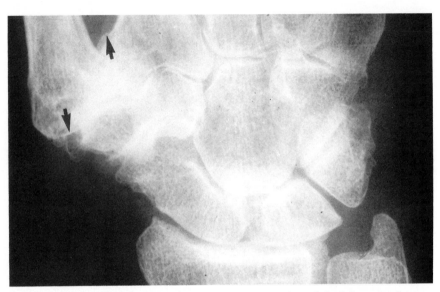

FIGURE 12–4. Osteoarthritis of the wrist. There is narrowing of the joint space between the base of the 1st metacarpal and the greater multangular and between the greater multangular and the navicular. There are subchondral sclerosis and osteophyte formation (arrows).

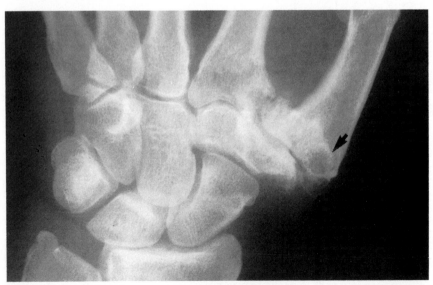

FIGURE 12–5. Osteoarthritis of the wrist. There is radial subluxation of the base of the 1st metacarpal in relationship to the greater multangular. There is associated subchondral sclerosis and osteophyte formation. A cyst is present in the base of the 1st metacarpal (arrow).

Erosive osteoarthritis is a close relative of primary osteoarthritis and should be discussed at this time. Erosive osteoarthritis is seen primarily in post-menopausal females. It has the same distribution in the hand that primary osteoarthritis has, with involvement of the DIP and PIP joints in the fingers (Fig. 12–6) and the 1st carpometacarpal joint and the greater multangular–navicular joint in the wrist (Fig. 12–7). It is distinguished from osteoarthritis in that it has an inflammatory component superimposed on osteoarthritic changes. Therefore, in addition to osteophyte formation, erosive disease is present and ankylosis can occur (Fig. 12–8). Occasionally confusion exists between erosive osteoarthritis and psoriasis. Psoriasis has no osteophyte formation and the erosions are marginal. Erosive osteoarthritis has osteophytes and the erosions are more central in location. Martel has likened the appearance of the erosive osteoarthritic joint to that of a "seagull" and the appearance of the psoriatic arthritic joint to that of "mouse ears" (Fig. 12–9). The only other joints involved with erosive osteoarthritis are the IP joints of the feet. The presence of erosions and osteophytes in any other joint in the body indicates an underlying inflammatory arthropathy with secondary osteoarthritis, not erosive osteoarthritis.

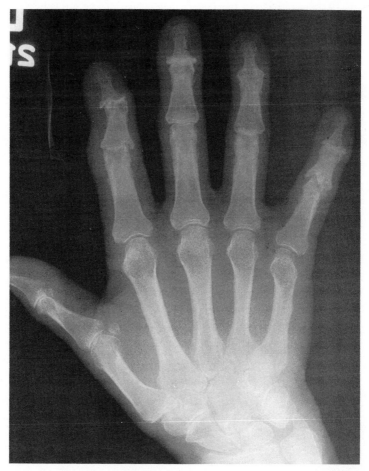

FIGURE 12–6. PA view of a hand with erosive osteoarthritis. Normal mineralization is present. There is involvement to varying degrees of all IP joints. The DIP joints show osteophyte formation. The 2nd and 5th PIP joints show erosive changes. The 5th PIP joint has the appearance of a "seagull." There is ankylosis of the 4th DIP joint.

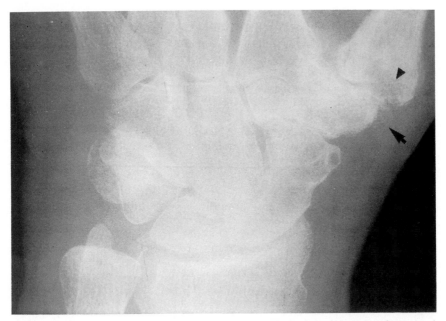

FIGURE 12–7. Wrist in erosive osteoarthritis. There is loss of the joint space between the base of the 1st metacarpal and the greater multangular. There are bone sclerosis and osteophyte formation (arrow). Erosive changes are seen in the base of the 1st metacarpal (arrowhead).

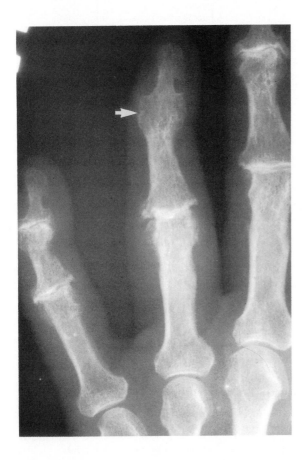

FIGURE 12–8. Erosive osteoarthritis involving the IP joints. Osteophyte formation is seen in all the IP joints. There is bone ankylosis of the 4th DIP joint (arrow) demonstrating the inflammatory component.

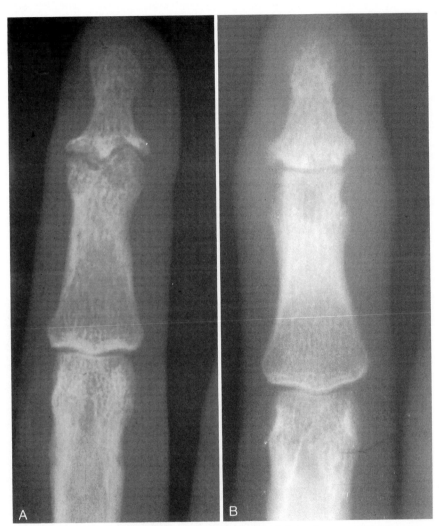

FIGURE 12–9. *A*, Erosive osteoarthritis involving the DIP joint demonstrating the appearance of a "seagull." *B*, Psoriatic arthritis of the DIP joint demonstrating the appearance of "mouse ears." (*B* from Brower AC: The radiographic features of psoriatic arthritis. *In* Gerger L, Espinoza L (eds): Psoriatic Arthritis. Orlando, FL, Grune & Stratton, Inc, 1985, p 125.)

THE FEET

The most common joint of the foot involved with osteoarthritis is the 1st MTP joint. This is usually seen in association with a hallux valgus or a hallux rigidus deformity of the big toe. There is non-uniform loss of the joint space. The sesamoids appear lateral to their normal relationship with the metatarsal head. Osteophyte formation, subchondral bone repair, and cyst formation are present (Fig. 12–10). There may be thickening of the lateral cortex of the 1st metatarsal as weight is placed on this area (Fig. 12–11). Osteoarthritic changes may be seen elsewhere in the foot wherever the normal mechanics are changed. For instance, a person with a tarsal coalition may develop osteoarthritis in the tarsal joints that are not congenitally fused.

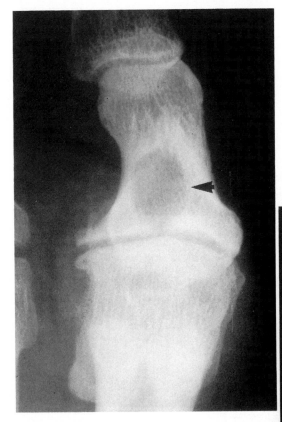

FIGURE 12–10. Osteoarthritis of the 1st MTP joint with hallux rigidus. There is loss of the joint space, subchondral sclerosis, and osteophyte formation. A subchondral cyst is seen in the base of the proximal phalanx (arrow).

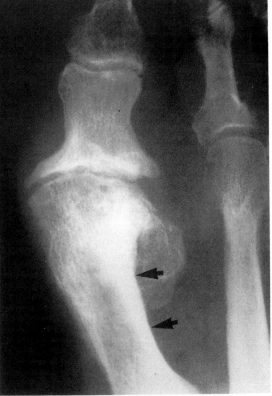

FIGURE 12–11. Osteoarthritis of the 1st MTP in a patient with a hallux valgus deformity. The sesamoids are lateral to the metatarsal head. There is narrowing of the joint space with subchondral bone and osteophyte formation. There is marked thickening of the lateral cortex of the metatarsal shaft (arrows).

THE HIPS

There is non-uniform loss of joint space in the hip joint which is radiographically identified as superolateral migration of the femoral head within the acetabulum (Fig. 12–12). If a vacuum phenomenon is produced within the joint, loss of cartilage is observed on the superolateral aspect of the hip joint, with maintenance of normal cartilage axially and medially (Fig. 12–13). As the cartilage is lost, subchondral bone formation and osteophyte formation are seen in this area of the joint (Fig. 12–12). With this cartilage loss and migration of the head within the acetabulum, the head becomes incongruous with the acetabulum. As a result, an osteophyte develops medially on the femoral head to fill the incongruity (Fig. 12–14). A ghost line of the original femoral head is often identified, with the osteophyte obviously being an addition to the head. The weight-bearing axis is shifted from its normal position to the medial neck of the femur, and new bone is added along the medial cortex (Fig. 12–12). Although there is no actual erosion as seen in the inflammatory arthropathies, there may be wearing away or grinding down of the bone on both sides of the joint, giving a nubbin appearance to the femoral head and a more vertical orientation to the acetabulum (Fig. 12–15).

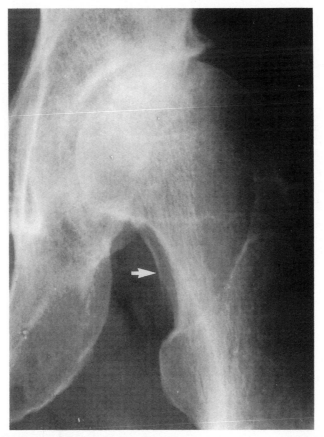

FIGURE 12–12. Osteoarthritis of the hip. There is non-uniform loss of the joint space with superolateral migration of the femoral head within the acetabulum. There are subchondral bone formation and an osteophyte seen on the lateral aspect of the acetabulum. There is new bone apposition along the medial cortex of the femoral neck (arrow). (From Brower AC: The radiologic approach to arthritis. Med Clin North Am 68:1593, 1984.)

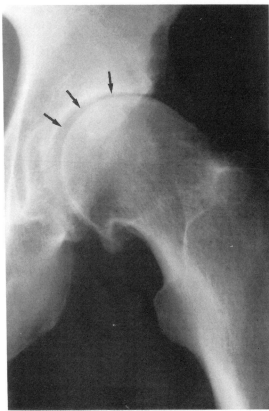

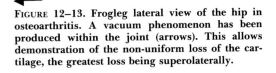

FIGURE 12–13. Frogleg lateral view of the hip in osteoarthritis. A vacuum phenomenon has been produced within the joint (arrows). This allows demonstration of the non-uniform loss of the cartilage, the greatest loss being superolaterally.

FIGURE 12–14. AP view of the hip in osteoarthritis. The hip has moved in a superolateral direction within the acetabulum. There is subchondral sclerosis, osteophyte formation, and cyst formation. A large osteophyte has been added to the medial aspect of the femoral head (arrows); it fills the incongruity between the acetabulum and the displaced head.

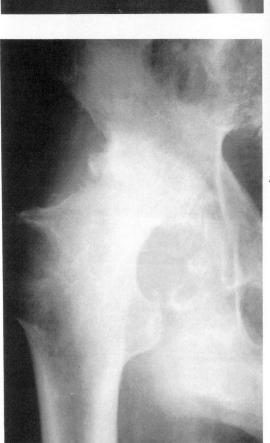

FIGURE 12–15. Severe osteoarthritis of the hip. The femoral head has been mechanically eroded to half its normal size. The acetabulum has been eroded to a more vertical orientation. There are extensive subchondral bone formation, osteophyte formation, and marked thickening of the inner cortex of the femoral neck.

Cyst formation is part of osteoarthritis. The cysts of osteoarthritis have been classified as *intrusion cysts* and *contusion cysts* (Fig. 12–16). The intrusion cyst is seen immediately subchondrally and may have a wide, narrow, or radiographically absent communication with the joint space. The contusion cyst may be further from the joint than the intrusion cyst and is totally enclosed within the bone. Both have sclerotic borders and reparative bone surrounding them. A cyst may collapse, producing a bizarre configuration of the femoral head. Cysts can also be present before there is actual cartilage loss and later cause secondary collapse of the joint.

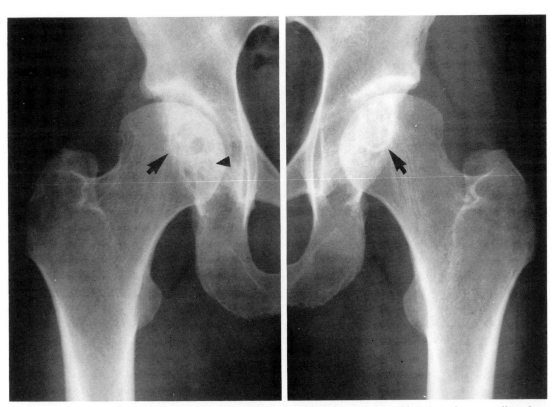

FIGURE 12–16. Cyst formation in osteoarthritis. In these hips there is no cartilage loss present. The intrusion cyst is seen immediately subchondrally (arrows), and the contusion cyst is seen further from the joint (arrowhead).

THE KNEES

Osteoarthritis of the knee is seen most commonly in the post-traumatic knee and in obese females. There is non-uniform loss of the joint space as manifested by preferential narrowing of the medial tibiofemoral compartment and the patellofemoral compartment (Fig. 12–17). There is a varus deformity in the standing knee, with lateral subluxation of the tibia in relationship to the femur. With this medial compartment loss and lateral subluxation, a large osteophyte forms on the medial aspect of the medial condyle (Fig. 12–18). Subchondral bone repair and cyst formation may be seen. There may be thickening of the medial cortex of the tibia as the axis of weight bearing is shifted to this area. Osteophyte formation and subchondral sclerosis develop in the posterior aspect of the tibia and the anterior aspect of the tibia and the femur (Fig. 12–19). Bone excrescences or exostoses may form and extend into the joint where cartilage has been lost (Fig. 12–20). Sometimes pieces of bone or cartilage break off and form loose bodies within the joint (Fig. 12–21). These changes should not be confused with primary synovial osteochondromatosis.

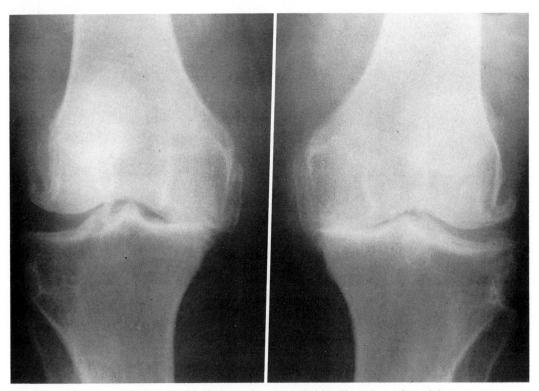

FIGURE 12–17. AP standing view of both knees in osteoarthritis. There is preferential narrowing of the medial tibiofemoral compartment with slight lateral subluxation of the tibia in relationship to the femur.

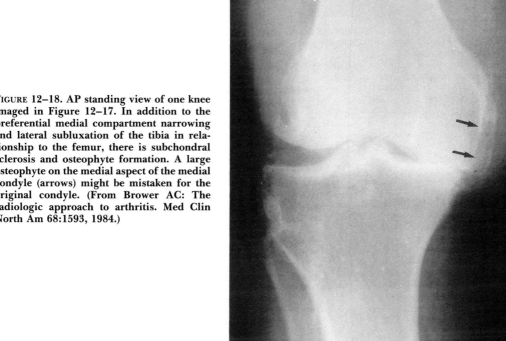

FIGURE 12–18. AP standing view of one knee imaged in Figure 12–17. In addition to the preferential medial compartment narrowing and lateral subluxation of the tibia in relationship to the femur, there is subchondral sclerosis and osteophyte formation. A large osteophyte on the medial aspect of the medial condyle (arrows) might be mistaken for the original condyle. (From Brower AC: The radiologic approach to arthritis. Med Clin North Am 68:1593, 1984.)

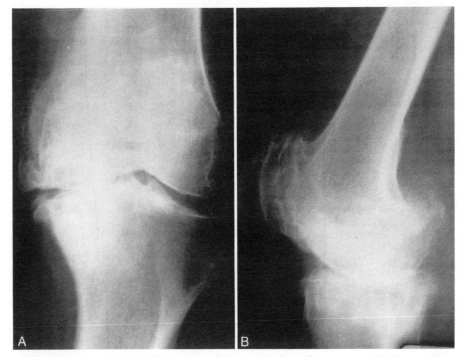

FIGURE 12–19. *A*, AP standing view and (*B*) lateral view of an osteoarthritic knee. There is preferential medial tibiofemoral and patellofemoral compartment narrowing. Varus deformity is noted on the AP view. There is extensive subchondral bone repair and osteophyte formation medially on the AP view and anteriorly and posteriorly on the lateral view.

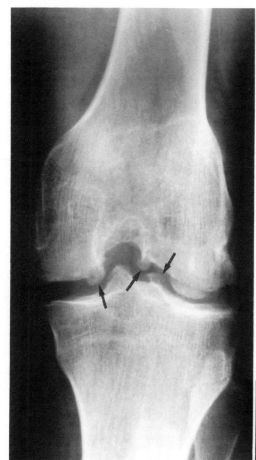

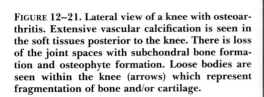

FIGURE 12–20. Tunnel view of a knee demonstrating bone excrescences extending into the joint from areas where cartilage has been lost (arrows).

FIGURE 12–21. Lateral view of a knee with osteoarthritis. Extensive vascular calcification is seen in the soft tissues posterior to the knee. There is loss of the joint spaces with subchondral bone formation and osteophyte formation. Loose bodies are seen within the knee (arrows) which represent fragmentation of bone and/or cartilage.

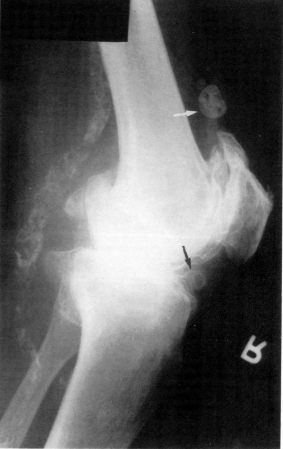

THE SACROILIAC JOINT

Osteoarthritis of the SI joint occurs most commonly in heavy laborers. The greatest loss of cartilage is seen in the superior and inferior aspects of the true synovial joint (Fig. 12–22). The loss is identified by the presence of subchondral bone repair. Osteophytes form superiorly and inferiorly and bridge across the ilium to the sacrum anteriorly. These osteophytes may be mistaken for bone ankylosis of the joint on an AP view. However, careful observation of a portion of the joint remaining unaffected should allow the correct diagnosis of osteoarthritis rather than inflammatory disease.

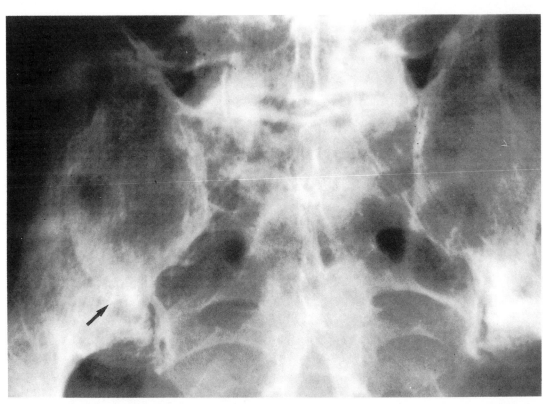

FIGURE 12–22. Sacroiliac joints in osteoarthritis. There is subchondral bone repair in the synovial aspect of the joint. Osteophytes extend from the ilium to the sacrum anteriorly (arrow); these should not be mistaken for ankylosis of the joint. (From Brower AC: Disorders of the sacroiliac joint. Radiolog 1(20):3, 1978.)

THE SPINE

Osteoarthritis of the spine means osteoarthritis of the apophyseal joints (Fig. 12–23). This is commonly seen in the lower lumbar spine and in the lower cervical spine. It is seen as narrowing of the apophyseal joints and bone sclerosis. Severe osteoarthritis allows grade I spondylolisthesis (Fig. 12–24) in the lumbar spine and minimal subluxation in the cervical spine.

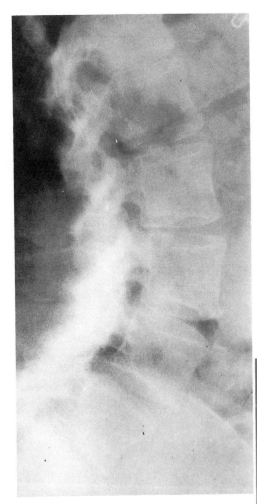

FIGURE 12–23. Lateral view of the lumbosacral spine showing osteoarthritis of the apophyseal joints. There is loss of the apophyseal joints with tremendous subchondral sclerosis present. The vertebral bodies and disc spaces are unaffected. (From Brower AC: The significance of the various phytes of the spine. Radiolog 1(15):3, 1978.)

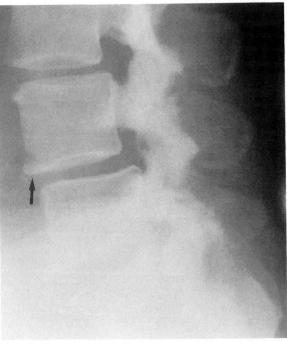

FIGURE 12–24. Lateral view of the lower lumbar spine with osteoarthritis. There is loss of the apophyseal joint spaces with adjacent subchondral sclerosis. There is a Grade I spondylolisthesis of L4 in relationship to L5 (arrow).

Narrowing and/or loss of disc height with osteophyte formation and subchondral bone sclerosis in the adjacent vertebral bodies should be called degenerative disc disease and not osteoarthritis. The disc is not a synovial joint and should not be attributed to a disease that primarily involves the synovial joints. Degenerative disc disease is seen most commonly in the lumbar spine at L4-L5 and L5-S1 and in the cervical spine at C5-C6 and C6-C7 (Fig. 12–25).

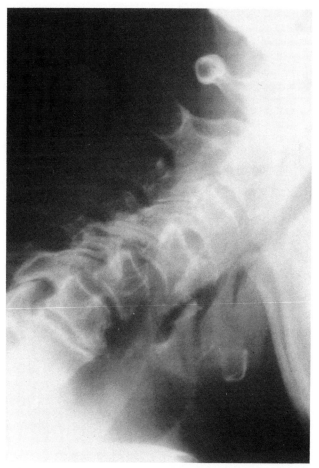

FIGURE 12–25. Lateral view of the cervical spine showing osteoarthritis of the apophyseal joints of the upper cervical spine. There is a resultant subluxation of C4 on C5. There is also degenerative disc disease present at C5-C6 and C6-C7. There is associated osteophyte formation at C6-C7, and there is subluxation of C5 on C6.

SUMMARY

The radiographic hallmarks of osteoarthritis are subchondral bone formation, osteophyte formation, and cysts. These changes may be seen secondary to a primary underlying arthropathy. In this instance the cartilage loss is uniform. However, if these radiographic findings occur with non-uniform loss of cartilage, the diagnosis must be primary osteoarthritis or osteoarthritis unrelated to a previous arthropathy.

SUGGESTED READINGS

Ahlback S: Osteoarthrosis of the knee. A radiographic investigation. Acta Radiol (Diagn) Suppl 277:7, 1968.

Cameron HU, Fornasier VL: Fine detail radiography of the femoral head in osteoarthritis. J Rheumatol 6:178, 1979.

Greenway G, Resnick D, Weisman M, Mink J: Carpal involvement in inflammatory (erosive) osteoarthritis. J Can Assoc Radiol 30:95, 1979.

Jeffery AK: Osteophytes and the osteoarthritic femoral head. J Bone Joint Surg 57B:314, 1975.

Kellgren JH, Lawrence JS, Bier F: Genetic factors in generalized osteoarthrosis. Ann Rheum Dis 22:237, 1963.

Kidd KL, Peter JB: Erosive osteoarthritis. Radiology 86:640, 1966.

Mann RA, Coughlin MJ, DuVries HL: Hallux rigidus. A review of the literature and a method of treatment. Clin Orthop Rel Res 142:57, 1979.

Martel W, Braunstein EM: The diagnostic value of buttressing of the femoral neck. Arthritis Rheum 21:161, 1978.

Martel W, Stuck Kj, Dworin AM, Hylland RG: Erosive osteoarthritis and psoriatic arthritis: A radiologic comparison in the hand, wrist, and foot. AJR 134:125, 1980.

Mitchell NS, Cruess RL: Classification of degenerative arthritis. Can Med Assoc J 117:763, 1977.

Murray RO: The aetiology of primary osteoarthritis of the hip. Br J Radiol 38:810, 1965.

Ondrouch AS: Cyst formation in osteoarthritis. J Bone Joint Surg 45B:755, 1963.

Resnick D: Patterns of migration of the femoral head in osteoarthritis of the hip. Roentgenographic-pathologic correlation and comparison with rheumatoid arthritis. AJR 124:62, 1975.

Resnick D, Niwayama G, Goergen TG: Degenerative disease of the sacroiliac joint. Invest Radiol 10:608, 1975.

Sims CD, Bentley G: Carpometacarpal osteoarthritis of the thumb. Br J Surg 57:442, 1970.

Thomas RH, Resnick D, Alazraki NP, et al.: Compartmental evaluation of osteoarthritis of the knee. A comparative study of available diagnostic modalities. Radiology 116:585, 1975.

Trueta J: Studies of the Development and Decay of the Human Frame. Philadelphia, W. B. Saunders Company, 1968, p 335.

chapter 13

NEUROPATHIC OSTEOARTHROPATHY

Neuropathic osteoarthropathy presents the most dramatic radiographic picture of all of the arthropathies. As a result, it may produce a diagnostic dilemma. While it is known that various neurological disorders play a prominent role in the development of the osteoarthropathy, the exact pathogenesis has not been clearly established. While chronic repetitive unsensed trauma creates many of the radiographic changes, it cannot be responsible for all of the changes seen. As long as trauma is believed to be the primary etiology, many neuropathic joints will continue to be misdiagnosed as infection or tumor.

The radiographic changes in neuropathic osteoarthropathy cover the complete spectrum of bone change from total resorption to excessive repair. At one end of the spectrum is the hypertrophic joint and at the other end the atrophic joint. Each of these extremes is discussed separately.

THE HYPERTROPHIC JOINT

The hypertrophic joint, or bone productive joint, if put in a time sequence, should be called the "chronic joint." The radiographic changes present no diagnostic problem. The changes resemble osteoarthritis "with a vengence." The hallmarks are the following:

1. **Dissolution of normal joint articulation**

2. **Severe subluxation and/or dislocation**

3. **Excessive juxta-articular new bone formation**

4. **Mammoth osteophytes**

5. Fragmentation and osseous debris

6. Pathological fractures

7. Unilateral or bilateral asymmetrical involvement

8. Distribution in weight-bearing joints, i.e., foot, ankle, knee, hip, spine

The Foot and Ankle

Today diabetes mellitus is the most common cause of neuropathic osteoarthropathy even though it occurs in only 5 to 10 per cent of diabetics. In diabetics the forefoot and midfoot are the most commonly involved joints. However, in diabetes, infection is commonly present and it becomes difficult to separate neuropathic changes from those of chronic osteomyelitis. The most common neuropathic change seen in the foot is radiographic evidence of a long-standing Lisfranc fracture-dislocation with extensive eburnation and fragmentation around the tarsometatarsal joints (Fig. 13–1). Bizarre fractures of the calcaneus with dissolution of the talocalcaneal joint and tumbling of the talus into the calcaneus may be the neuropathic change (Fig. 13–2). In the ankle, the distal fibula may fracture pathologically and the talus angulate within the ankle mortise. With time, massive bone sclerosis, osteophytosis, and osseous debris develop (Fig. 13–3).

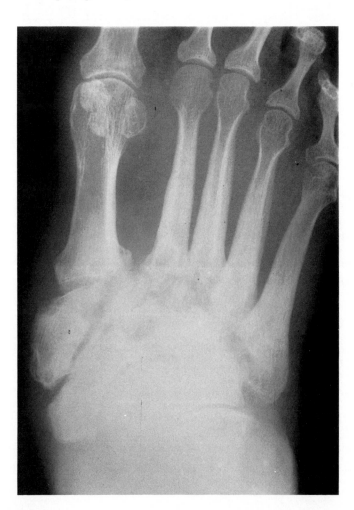

FIGURE 13–1. AP view of the forefoot in a diabetic patient. There is a Lisfranc fracture-dislocation of the tarsometatarsal joints. There is extensive subchondral sclerosis in the adjacent articulating bones.

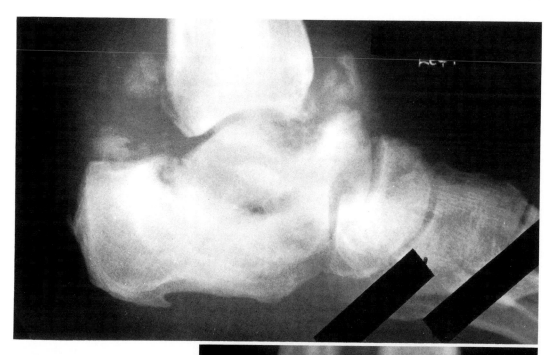

FIGURE 13–2. A lateral view of the hindfoot in a diabetic patient. There is dissolution of the talocalcaneal joint space, with the talus tumbling into the calcaneus. There is extensive subchondral bone formation. Fragments of bone are seen in the ankle joint. (From Brower AC, Allman RM: Neuropathic osteoarthropathy in the adult. *In* Traveras JM, Ferruci JT (eds): Radiology: Diagnosis/Imaging/Intervention. Vol. 5. Philadelphia, J. B. Lippincott, 1986.)

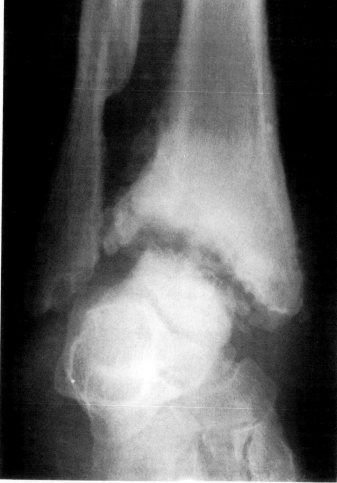

FIGURE 13–3. AP view of a neuropathic ankle. There is complete dissolution of the normal ankle joint. There is extensive subchondral sclerosis in both the tibia and adjacent talus. There is fragmentation within the joint space. An old healed fracture of the distal shaft of the fibula is evident.

Knee and Hip

These joints are most commonly involved in tabes dorsalis. Sixty to 70 per cent of patients with this condition have lower extremity involvement. In the knee the first radiographic change is recurrent massive effusion with some subluxation. Periarticular pathological fractures and bone debris within the joint may develop (Fig. 13–4). Eventually with weight bearing there is joint dissolution, subluxation, eburnation, and fragmentation (Fig. 13–5).

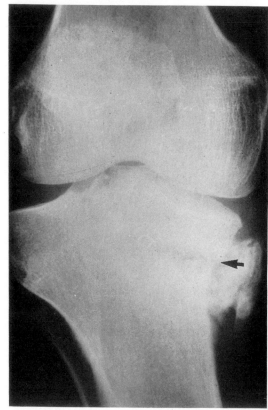

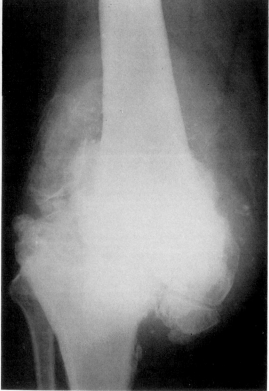

FIGURE 13–4. AP view of a neuropathic knee showing a pathological transverse fracture just beneath the lateral tibial plateau (arrow). Excess ossification is seen adjacent to this. The tibia is subluxed laterally in relationship to the femur. (From Brower AC, Allman RM: The pathogenesis of the neurotropic joint: Neurotraumatic vs. neurovascular. Radiology 139:349–354, 1981.)

FIGURE 13–5. AP view of a neuropathic knee showing total dissolution of the joint space, extensive subluxation, massive subchondral sclerosis, and fragmentation. (From Brower AC, Allman RM: The neuropathic joint—A neurovascular bone disorder. Radiol Clin North Am 19:571–580, 1981.)

The early changes described in the knee are more difficult to observe in the hip. If the patient is weight bearing, productive bone changes develop around the femoral head and a pseudoacetabulum is formed where the head has subluxed from the normal acetabulum (Fig. 13–6).

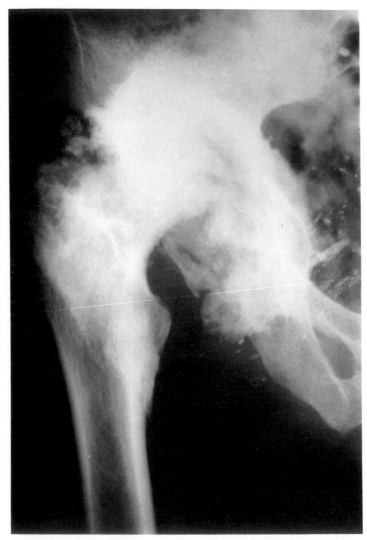

FIGURE 13–6. AP view of a neuropathic hip. The superior portion of the acetabulum has become eroded and remodeled, forming a large shallow pseudo-acetabulum. There is massive bone formation in both the acetabulum and the femoral head. Osteophytosis and fragmentation are present as well.

The Spine

While spine involvement is most commonly associated with tabes dorsalis, it may be observed in diabetes. One or several disc levels and the adjacent vertebral bodies may be involved. The radiographic picture is one of bizarre and extreme degenerative disc disease (Fig. 13–7). Eventually there is complete dissolution of the normal disc space, with massive sclerosis and excessive osteophytosis of the adjacent vertebral bodies (Fig. 13–8). Bone fragmentation, although present, may be difficult to observe. One vertebral body appears to be tumbling into the adjacent vertebral body (Fig. 13–9).

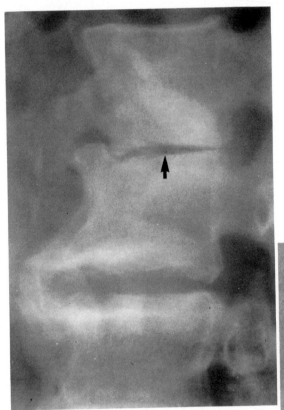

◄

FIGURE 13–7. A lateral view of three lumbar vertebral bodies. A vacuum phenomenon is present at the upper disc level (arrow). The superior vertebral body is tumbling into the inferior vertebral body. There is sclerosis involving half of the upper vertebral body and one third of the lower vertebral body. Although the changes resemble degenerative disc disease, the bone formation is more extensive and the tumbling of one vertebral body into an adjacent vertebral body is unusual for uncomplicated degenerative disc disease.

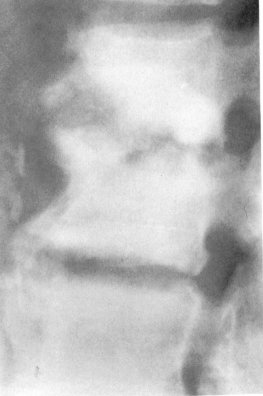

FIGURE 13–8. Lateral view of the lumbar spine shown in Figure 13–7 one year later. There is complete dissolution of the disc space, with massive eburnation in the adjacent vertebral bodies along with osteophyte formation.

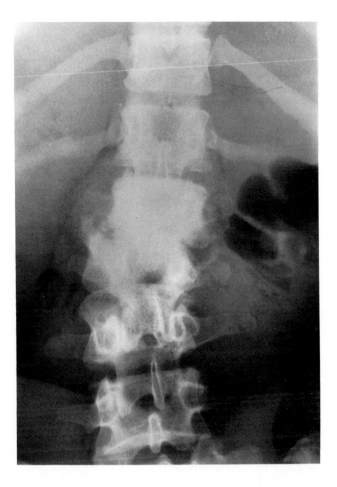

FIGURE 13–9. AP view of the upper lumbar spine in a patient with diabetes. L1 appears to be tumbling into L2. There is no evidence of a remaining disc space. Both vertebral bodies have become completely sclerotic. (From Brower AC, Allman RM: Neuropathic osteoarthropathy in the adults. *In* Traveras JM, Ferruci JT (eds): Radiology: Diagnosis/Imaging/Intervention. Vol 5. Philadelphia, J. B. Lippincott, 1986.)

THE ATROPHIC JOINT

The atrophic or resorbed joint, if put in a time sequence, should be called the "acute joint." In this type of neuropathic joint, radiographs reveal change from normal to dramatic resorption within a period of three to four weeks. The radiographic appearance is often mistaken for a rampant infection or an aggressive bone tumor. The radiographic hallmarks are the following:

1. Extensive bone resorption

2. Sharp edge, resembling surgical amputation, between resorbed bone and remaining bone

3. Normal mineralization in remaining bone

4. Absence of bone repair

5. Soft tissue swelling

6. Bone debris in soft tissue

7. Unilateral or bilateral asymmetrical involvement

8. Distribution in non–weight-bearing joints, shoulder and elbow predominantly; also seen in a non–weight-bearing hip and knee

The Shoulder and Elbow

The most common cause of neuropathic osteoarthropathy in the shoulder and elbow is syringomyelia. Twenty to 25 per cent of patients with syringomyelia develop a neuropathic joint. In either the shoulder or elbow joint, soft tissue swelling is seen, with osseous debris within it. Varying degrees of resorption of the articulating bones can be identified. The remaining ends of the bones appear to be surgically amputated (Figs. 13–10 to 13–12). In the shoulder pathological fractures may be seen in the adjacent scapula or acromion (Fig. 13–13).

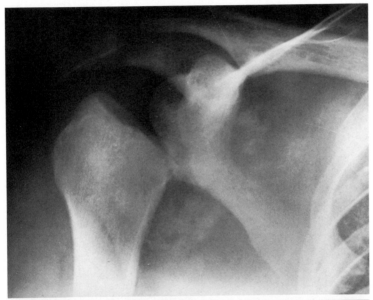

FIGURE 13–10. AP view of the shoulder in syringomyelia. Part of the humeral head has been totally resorbed. There is a sharp edge to the remaining bone, giving the appearance of a surgical amputation. Debris is seen within the joint. (From Brower AC, Allman RM: Neuropathic osteoarthropathy in the adult. In Traveras JM, Ferruci JT (eds): Radiology: Diagnosis/Imaging/Intervention. Vol. 5. Philadelphia, J. B. Lippincott, 1986.)

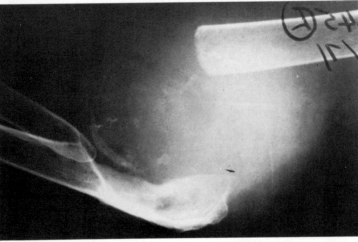

FIGURE 13–11. A lateral view of an elbow in syringomyelia. There is tremendous soft tissue swelling in the area of the elbow joint. Ossific debris is seen within the soft tissue swelling. The proximal end of the radius appears whittled. The proximal end of the ulna is shallowed out, and the distal end of the humerus has a sharp, surgical-appearing edge. Changes are classic for an atrophic neuropathic joint. (From Brower AC, Allman RM: The neuropathic joint—A neurovascular bone disorder. Radiol Clin North Am 19:571–580, 1981.)

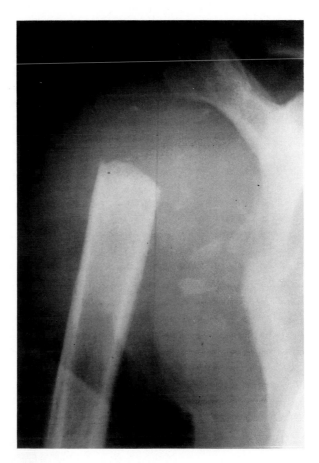

FIGURE 13–12. AP view of the shoulder in syringomyelia. Soft tissue swelling is present in the area of the previous shoulder joint. Ossific debris is seen within the soft tissue. All of the humeral head and part of the proximal shaft have been resorbed. The remaining humerus is normally mineralized and has a sharp, surgical-appearing edge. (From Brower AC, Allman RM: The pathogenesis of the neurotrophic joint: Neurotraumatic vs. neurovascular. Radiology 139:349–354, 1981.)

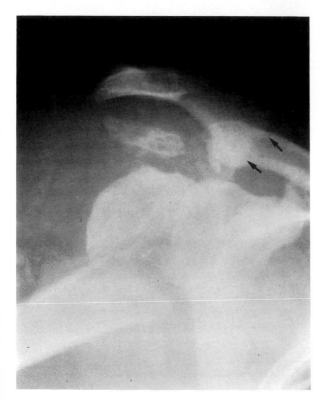

FIGURE 13–13. AP view of the shoulder in syringomyelia. Half of the humeral head has been resorbed. The remaining humeral head is fractured from the remaining shaft. The acromion has been pathologically fractured from the scapula (arrows). Ossific debris is present within the joint. (From Brower AC, Allman RM: The pathogenesis of the neurotrophic joint: Neurotraumatic vs. neurovascular. Radiology 139:349–354, 1981.)

The Hip

In the non–weight-bearing hip (e.g., in a paraplegic), there are varying degrees of extensive resorption of the femoral head with a surgical sharp edge to the remaining bone (Fig. 13–14). Osseous debris is seen in the joint space. The hip may sublux laterally and superiorly to the acetabulum. After considerable time has passed, as long as the patient continues not to bear weight on the hip, a cortical border forms at the surgical edge of the resorbed bone. The acetabulum remodels to accommodate the subluxed hip (Fig. 13–15). The osseous debris becomes well-corticated bone fragments. However, the massive subchondral sclerosis and osteophytosis seen in a weight-bearing neuropathic hip does not occur.

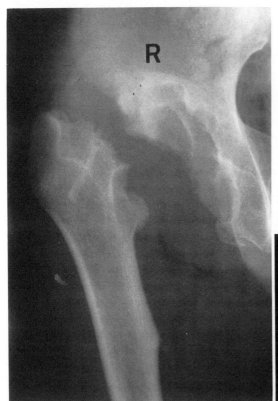

←

FIGURE 13–14. AP view of an atrophic neuropathic hip. There has been complete resorption of the femoral head and most of the femoral neck. There has been some resorption and shallowing out of the acetabulum. There is a sharp edge to the remaining femur. The femur is subluxed laterally and superiorly to the acetabulum. (From Brower AC, Allman RM: Neuropathic osteoarthropathy in the adult. *In* Traveras JM, Ferruci JT (eds): Radiology: Diagnosis/Imaging/Intervention. Vol 5. Philadelphia, J. B. Lippincott, 1986.)

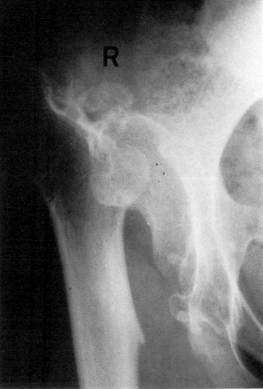

FIGURE 13–15. AP view of the same hip shown in Figure 13–14 three years later. The femoral head and neck are absent. The remaining femoral shaft and adjacent acetabulum are well corticated. Bone fragments within the joint have become well corticated. There is absence of massive subchondral sclerosis and osteophytosis. (From Brower AC, Allman RM: Neuropathic osteoarthropathy in the adult. *In* Traveras JM, Ferruci JT (eds): Radiology: Diagnosis/Imaging/Intervention. Vol 5. Philadelphia, J. B. Lippincott, 1986.)

COMBINED HYPERTROPHY AND ATROPHY

While the hypertrophic and atrophic joints represent the extremes of neuropathic osteoarthropathy, there are a large number of neuropathic joints that present with a combination of both bone resorption and bone production (Fig. 13–16). A segment of bone may be totally absent, while the remaining bone shows eburnation, fragmentation, and osteophytosis. Therefore in the diabetic ankle and foot, one should be careful of interpreting this combination of resorption and production as infection. It must be recognized that the neuropathic joint goes through a spectrum of changes that are directly related to the amount of weight the joint bears.

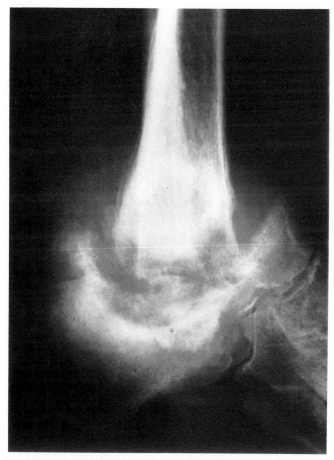

FIGURE 13–16. A lateral view of a neuropathic ankle. There is complete dissolution of the tibiotalar joint. Most of the talus has been resorbed, as well as a portion of the calcaneus. The remaining calcaneus and the anterior portion of the talus show massive subchondral sclerosis and osteophytosis. There is also massive subchondral sclerosis present in the distal tibia with some osteophytosis. This ankle represents the combination of bone resorption and production. (From Brower AC, Allman RM: The pathogenesis of the neurotrophic joint: Neurotraumatic vs. neurovascular. Radiology 139:349–354, 1981.)

SUMMARY

Neuropathic osteoarthropathy is a dramatic arthropathy that is both easily diagnosed and easily misdiagnosed. It presents the spectrum of bone changes from extensive resorption to excessive production.

SUGGESTED READINGS

Brower A, Allman RM: The neuropathic joint: A neurovascular bone disorder. Radiol Clin North Am 19:571, 1981.

Delano PJ: The pathogenesis of Charcot's joint. AJR 56:189, 1946.

Feldman F: Neuropathic osteoarthropathy. *In* Margulis AR, Gooding CA (eds.): Diagnostic Radiology. San Francisco, University of California Press, 1977, p 397.

Johnson JTH: Neuropathic fractures and joint injuries. Pathogenesis and rationale of prevention and treatment. J Bone Joint Surg 49A:1, 1967.

Johnson LC: Circulation and bone (Charcot's disease and trophic change). *In* Frost HM (ed.): Bone Biodynamics. Boston, Little, Brown and Company, 1964, p 603.

Katz I, Rabinowitz JG, Dziadiw R: Early changes in Charcot's joints. AJR 86:965, 1961.

Norman A, Robbins H, Milgram JE: The acute neuropathic arthropathy—a rapid, severely disorganizing form of arthritis. Radiology 90:1159, 1968.

chapter 14

DIFFUSE IDIOPATHIC SKELETAL HYPEROSTOSIS (DISH)

Diffuse idiopathic skeletal hyperostosis (DISH), also known as anky-losing hyperostosis or Forestier's disease, is not an arthropathy. The articular cartilage, adjacent bone margins, and synovium are not affected. DISH appears to be a bone-forming diathesis in which ossification occurs at skeletal sites subjected to stress, primarily at tendinous and ligamentous attachments. It is a common disorder, occurring in 12 per cent of the elderly population. Its radiographic manifestations have been mistaken for ankylosing spondylitis, other spondyloarthropathies, and osteoarthritis. Although it may coexist with an arthropathy, it should not be mistaken for a manifestation of that arthropathy. Knowledge of the radiographic criteria allows the correct diagnosis to be made. The radiographic findings are the following:

1. **Normal mineralization**

2. **Flowing ossification of at least four contiguous vertebral bodies**

3. **Preservation of disc spaces**

4. **Ossification of multiple tendinous and ligamentous sites in the appendicular skeleton**

5. Absence of joint abnormality

6. Sporadic distribution

7. Distribution primarily in the spine

The radiographic manifestations of DISH divide into those associated with the spine and those that are extraspinal. Extraspinal changes without spinal involvement are possible but extremely unusual.

SPINAL MANIFESTATIONS

Ossification of the ligaments and soft tissues that surround the vertebral bodies occurs. This must be observed around four or more contiguous vertebral bodies in order to make the diagnosis of DISH. The thickness of the ossification can range from 1 to 20 mm. Bone excrescences of various shapes may be observed. The ossification may be so extensive as to render the spine as immobile as one with ankylosing spondylitis.

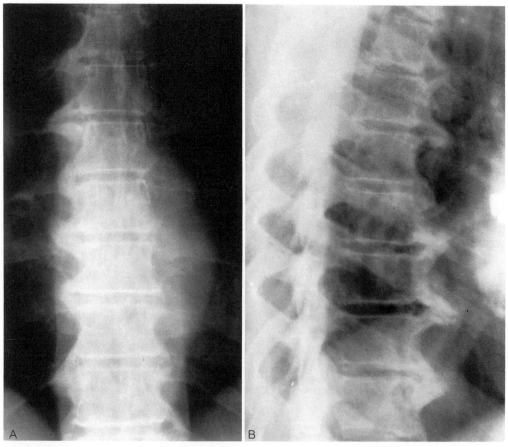

FIGURE 14–1. AP (A) and lateral (B) views of the thoracic spine in DISH. Flowing ossification is noted anteriorly and on the right side of the spine. At least seven contiguous vertebral bodies are involved. The disc spaces are preserved. Radiolucency extends from the disc space into the ossification, creating a Y-shaped lucency and a bumpy bone excrescence at the disc level. (B from Brower AC: The significance of the various phytes of the spine. Radiolog 1(15):3, 1978.)

The Thoracic Spine

The thoracic spine is the most common site of involvement. Flowing ossification is observed here in 97 to 100 per cent of patients with DISH. It is usually seen anteriorly and/or on the right side in the lower thoracic spine, from T7 to T11 (Fig. 14–1). The thickness of the ossification can range from 1 or 2 mm to 20 mm. It may be smooth or bumpy in contour, depending upon the configuration of the bone excrescences at the disc levels. The radiolucent disc may appear to protrude into the flowing ossification, creating an L-, T-, or Y-shaped defect at the disc level (Fig. 14–2). If the flowing ossification is thin and smooth, it may be mistaken for the ossification seen in ankylosing spondylitis (Fig. 14–3). Usually at some point a lucent line separates the flowing ossification from the adjacent vertebral body and thus distinguishes DISH from ankylosing spondylitis (Fig. 14–4).

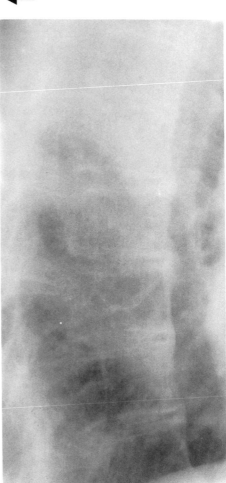

FIGURE 14–2. Lateral view of the lower thoracic spine in DISH. Lucency separates the flowing ossification from the adjacent vertebral body (arrow). Lucent defects are seen in the bony excrescences at the disc level, creating a T-shaped defect (arrowhead).

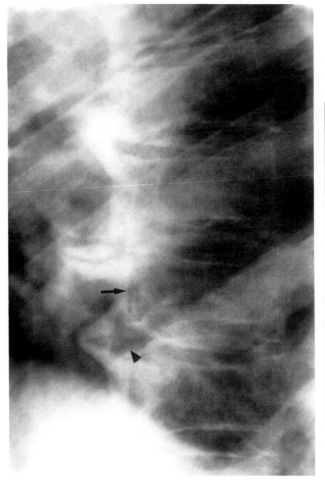

FIGURE 14–3. Lateral view of the lower thoracic spine involved with DISH. The flowing ossification is thin and smooth, resembling that of ankylosing spondylitis.

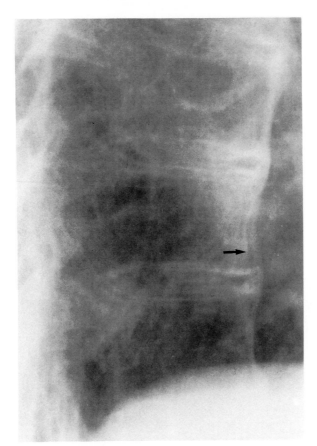

Figure 14-4. Close-up view of three thoracic vertebral bodies seen in Figure 14-3. A lucent line separates the flowing ossification from the adjacent vertebral body (arrow), establishing the diagnosis of DISH rather than ankylosing spondylitis.

The Cervical Spine

The cervical spine is involved in 78 per cent of patients with DISH. The abnormalities seen are most common in the lower cervical region. The flowing ossification anteriorly can vary from 1 to 12 mm in thickness. It may be very smooth in contour and appear to be an extension of the anterior border of the vertebral body (Fig. 14-5). It may be very bumpy, with the bumps occurring at the disc levels (Fig. 14-6). The ossification may impinge upon the esophagus, causing dysphagia (Fig. 14-7). The disc heights are preserved and the apophyseal joints are uninvolved. In some patients the posterior longitudinal ligament may be ossified, creating spinal stenosis.

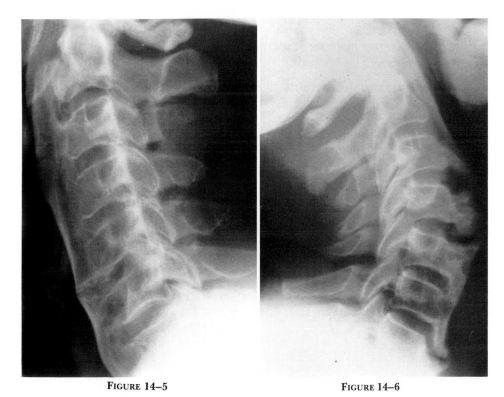

FIGURE 14–5   FIGURE 14–6

FIGURE 14–5. Lateral view of the cervical spine in DISH. There is thick but smooth ossification anterior to the vertebral bodies. The disc spaces are preserved. The apophyseal joints are uninvolved.

FIGURE 14–6. Lateral view of the cervical spine with DISH. There is thick, bumpy ossification anterior to the vertebral bodies. The disc spaces are maintained and the apophyseal joints are uninvolved.

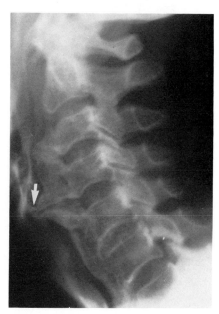

FIGURE 14–7. Lateral view of the cervical spine in DISH. There is excessive flowing ossification anterior to the vertebral bodies. Barium introduced into the esophagus allows demonstration of impingement on the esophagus by the ossification (arrow). The disc spaces are maintained. The apophyseal joints are uninvolved.

The Lumbar Spine

The lumbar spine is involved in 93 per cent of patients with DISH. The ossification may be more profound than that seen in the thoracic or cervical spine (Fig. 14–8). Some patients show flowing ossification similar to that seen in the thoracic spine (Fig. 14–9). Others show huge bony protuberances or excrescences primarily at the disc levels, resembling excessive osteophytosis (Fig. 14–10). However, the disc space is usually maintained and the apophyseal joints are uninvolved. Although DISH usually protects the patient from degenerative disc disease, it is possible for a patient to have both. Nevertheless, the two disorders should be recognized as separate entities so that the cause of clinical symptoms can be correctly addressed.

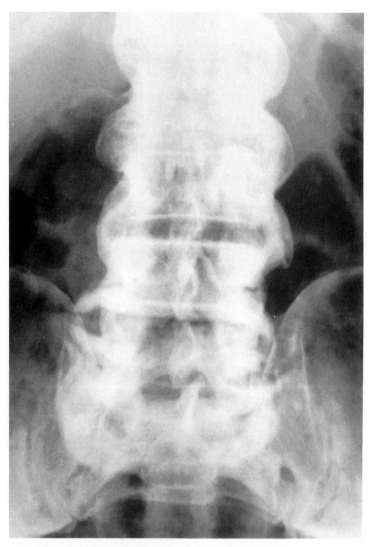

FIGURE 14–8. AP view of the lumbosacral spine in DISH. There is excessive flowing ossification bilaterally encasing the vertebral bodies and disc spaces. The discs are preserved. The sacroiliac joints are normal. (From Brower AC: The significance of the various phytes of the spine. Radiolog 1(15):3, 1978.)

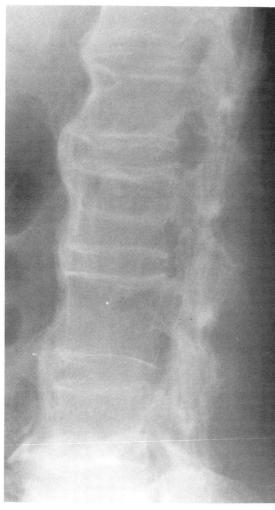

FIGURE 14–9. Lateral view of the lumbar spine in DISH. There is flowing smooth ossification anterior to the vertebral bodies. The disc spaces are preserved. The apophyseal joints are not involved.

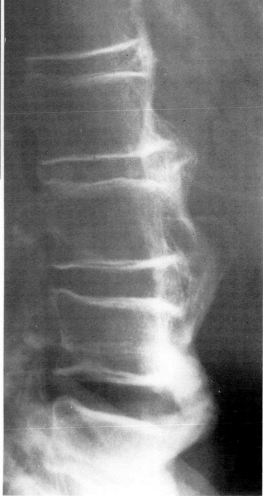

FIGURE 14–10. Lateral view of the lumbar spine in DISH. There is excessive bone formation anterior to the vertebral bodies, with huge bony excrescences at the disc levels. The discs are maintained.

EXTRASPINAL MANIFESTATIONS

The extraspinal radiographic manifestation of DISH is ossification of tendons and ligaments, predominantly at sites of attachment. While such ossification occurs in the "normal" population, the number of sites is usually limited. In DISH, this ossification occurs at multiple sites. This ossification may be misinterpreted as osteophytosis in osteoarthritis. However, in DISH there is no radiographic change in the joint itself.

The Pelvis

One hundred per cent of patients with extraspinal DISH have pelvic involvement. There is whiskering of the iliac crests, the ischial tuberosities, and the femoral trochanters (Fig. 14–11) similar to that seen in the spondyloarthropathies. Lack of involvement of the true synovial part of the sacroiliac joint distinguishes DISH from the spondyloarthropathies. Although DISH does not affect the synovial aspect of the sacroiliac joint, it may affect the rest of the joint. The posterior superior segment of the sacroiliac joint is not a joint, but a ligamentous bridge between the two bones. In DISH this area may ossify. There may also be ossification across the superior aspect of the pubic symphysis (Fig. 14–12). Although the hip joint itself is preserved, bone excrescences may form at the acetabular margins (Fig. 14–13).

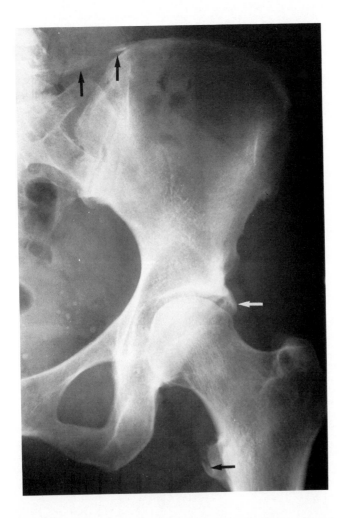

FIGURE 14–11. AP view of the left pelvis in DISH. There is ossification of the lesser trochanter, the lateral acetabular margin, and the iliac crest extending toward the transverse process of L5 (arrows). The hip joint is preserved.

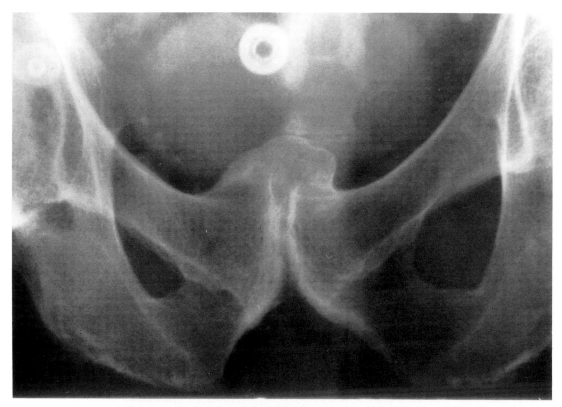

FIGURE 14–12. Pubic symphysis in DISH. There is ossification bridging the pubic rami superiorly.

FIGURE 14–13. AP view of the hip in DISH. Bone excrescences are seen at the margins of the acetabulum. The hip joint is maintained. There is ossification of the trochanters as well.

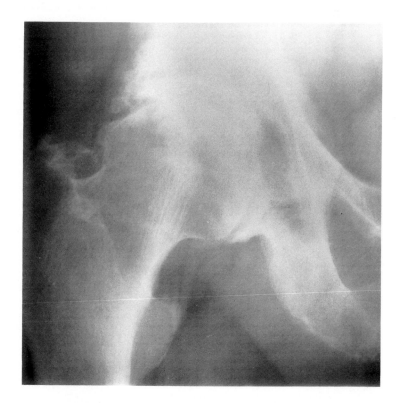

The Foot

Ossification is seen on the calcaneus in 75 per cent of the patients with extraspinal DISH. This ossification occurs at the Achilles tendon and the plantar aponeurosis (Fig. 14–14). The ossification may become quite extensive; it may then fracture, resulting in disruption of the tendon. The common locations for ossification in the rest of the foot are the dorsal aspect of the talus, the dorsal and medial aspects of the tarsal navicular, the lateral and plantar aspects of the cuboid, and the lateral aspect of the base of the 5th metatarsal (Fig. 14–15).

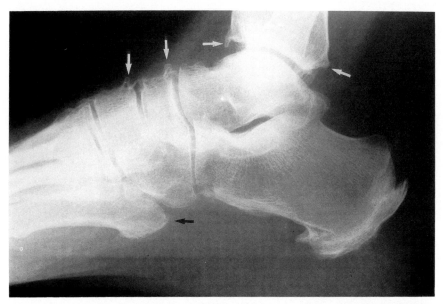

FIGURE 14–14. Lateral view of the foot in DISH. All joint spaces are preserved. Ossification is seen at the attachment of the plantar aponeurosis and the Achilles tendon. There is also ossification on the dorsal aspect of the navicular and the cuneiform, the base of the 5th metatarsal, and the distal tibia (arrows).

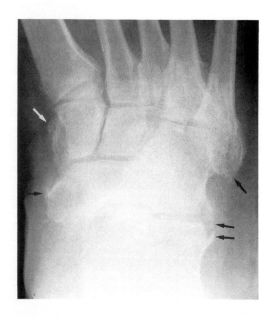

FIGURE 14–15. AP view of the foot shows ossification lateral to the calcaneus, the cuboid, and the base of the 5th metatarsal and medial to the navicular and the cuneiform (arrows).

The Knee

Ossification around the knee occurs in 29 per cent of patients with extraspinal DISH. It is most commonly seen in the inferior and superior patellar tendon (Fig. 14–16). The anterior portion of the patella itself may have irregular new bone apposition. There may be ossification of the tibial tubercle in a fashion suggestive of Osgood-Schlatter's disease. The medial collateral ligament ossifies, similar to Pellegrini-Stieda syndrome.

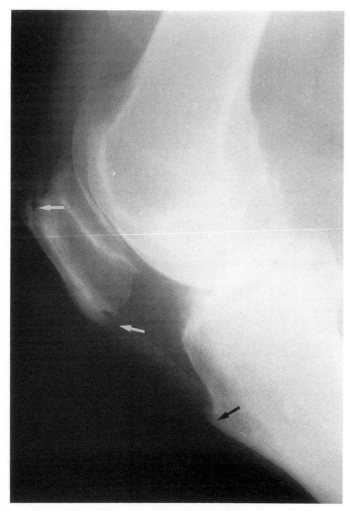

FIGURE 14–16. Lateral view of the knee in DISH. Ossification is seen of the superior and inferior patellar tendon as well as the tibial tubercle (arrows).

The Elbow

Ossification around the elbow occurs in 49 per cent of patients with extraspinal DISH. Spurring of the olecranon is the most common ossification. Around the elbow ossification may become so extensive as to be misdiagnosed as osteoarthritis (Fig. 14–17). Absence of true joint changes should prevent the clinician from making a diagnosis of osteoarthritis. The correct diagnosis is important in the treatment of the patient, who may have limited range of motion in the elbow secondary to this ossification.

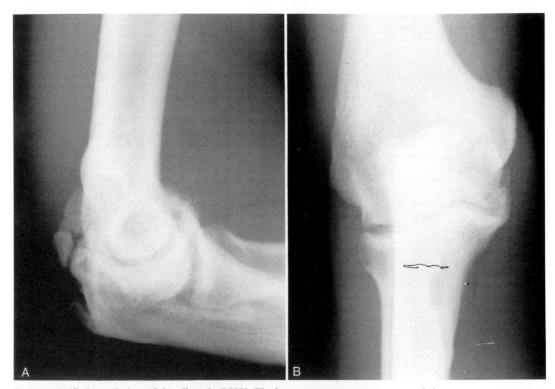

FIGURE 14–17. Lateral view of the elbow in DISH. The bone excrescences seen around the elbow resemble the osteophytes of osteoarthritis. *B*, AP view of the same elbow shows that the joint is preserved. There is no subchondral sclerosis or cyst formation. The bone excrescences are ossified tendinous attachments. (*A* from Brower AC: The significance of the various phytes of the spine. Radiolog 1(15):3, 1978.)

Other Sites

Ossification may occur in any ligamentous attachment. Other common sites are the deltoid protuberance on the humerus, the coracoclavicular ligament, the posterior superior aspect of the femur, and the shafts of the phalanges (Fig. 14–18).

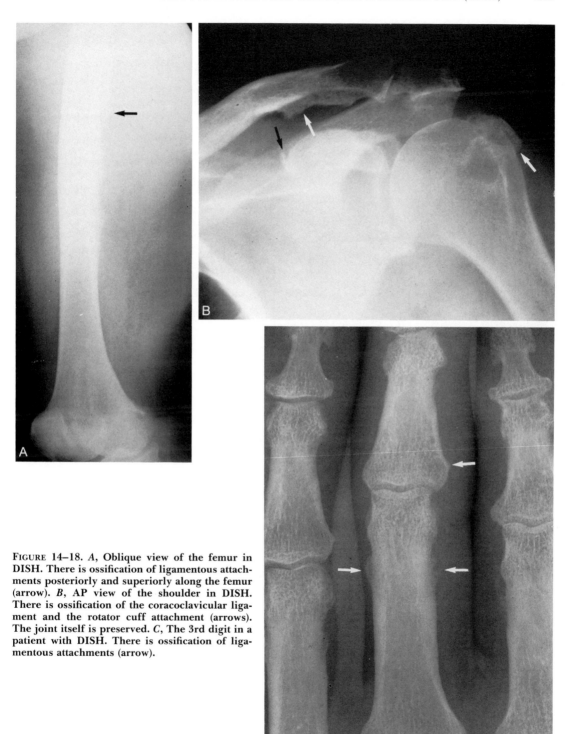

FIGURE 14–18. *A*, Oblique view of the femur in DISH. There is ossification of ligamentous attachments posteriorly and superiorly along the femur (arrow). *B*, AP view of the shoulder in DISH. There is ossification of the coracoclavicular ligament and the rotator cuff attachment (arrows). The joint itself is preserved. *C*, The 3rd digit in a patient with DISH. There is ossification of ligamentous attachments (arrow).

SUMMARY

DISH is not an arthropathy but a bone-forming diathesis. It will not be misdiagnosed as an arthropathy if two observations are made: (1) The ossification present is in ligamentous and tendinous sites, and (2) the disc space and/or the joint space is preserved.

SUGGESTED READINGS

Forestier J, Lagier R: Ankylosing hyperostosis of the spine. Clin Orthop 74:65–83, 1971.

Forestier J, Rotes-Querol J: Senile ankylosing hyperostosis of the spine. Ann Rheum Dis 9:321–330, 1950.

Resnick D, Guerra J, Robinson C, Vint V: Association of diffuse idiopathic skeletal hyperostosis (DISH) and calcification and ossification of the posterior longitudinal ligament. AJR 131:1049–1053, 1978.

Resnick D, Niwayama G: Radiographic and pathologic features of spinal involvement in diffuse idiopathic skeletal hyperostosis (DISH). Radiology 119:559–568, 1976.

Resnick D, Shapiro R, Wiesner K, et al: Diffuse idiopathic skeletal hyperostosis (DISH) (ankylosing hyperostosis of Forestier and Rotes-Querol). Semin Arthritis Rheum 7:153–187, 1978.

Resnick D, Shaul SR, Robins JM: Diffuse idiopathic skeletal hyperostosis (DISH): Forestier's disease with extraspinal manifestations. Radiology 115:513–524, 1975.

Sutro CJ, Ehrlich DE, Witten M: Generalized juxta-articular ossification of ligaments of the vertebral column and of the ligamentous and tendinous tissues of the extremities (also known as Bechterew's disease, osteophytosis and spondylosis deformans). Bull Hosp Joint Dis 17:343–357, 1956.

chapter *15*

GOUT

Gout is the oldest recognized arthropathy. It was originally called podagra, from the Greek *pous*, meaning foot, and *agra*, meaning attack. In ancient history all arthritis was called gout. Today we know it to be a specific arthropathy secondary to deposition of monosodium urate crystals. It occurs in 0.3 per cent of the population. Today it accounts for 5 per cent of all patients with arthritis. It is predominantly a disorder of males, occurring 20 times more frequently than in females. When it occurs in females, it is in the post-menopausal female.

There are two types of gout: (1) primary idiopathic gout due to an inborn error of metabolism, leading to the increase in uric acid in the blood, and (2) secondary gout associated with various diseases that cause increased production and/or decreased excretion of uric acid. Secondary gout does not usually produce radiographic changes.

Only 45 per cent of patients with gout manifest radiographic bone changes, and then only six to eight years after the initial attack. The radiographic changes indicate the chronicity of the disease process. Urate crystals deposit in tissues with poor blood supply: cartilage, tendon sheaths, bursa, etc. The radiographic presentation is dependent upon where the urate crystals are deposited. If they are deposited in cartilage, the radiographic picture will be that of osteoarthritis; if they are deposited in soft tissue, it will be that of chronic tophaceous gout. The hallmarks of osteoarthritis are discussed elsewhere. The radiographic features of chronic tophaceous gout are as follows:

1. **Tophi**

2. **Normal mineralization**

3. **Joint space preservation**

4. **Punched-out erosions with sclerotic borders**

5. Overhanging edge of cortex

6. Asymmetrical polyarticular distribution

7. Distribution in feet, ankles, knees, hands, and elbows in decreasing order of frequency

Since the radiographic features of chronic tophaceous gout are pathognomonic of the disease no matter what joint is involved, the features are discussed in greater detail before describing the distribution. It must be remembered that osteoarthritis developing secondary to urate crystal deposition in cartilage cannot be distinguished from osteoarthritis secondary to any other etiology. One must rely on the radiographic findings of tophaceous deposit.

Tophi are soft tissue masses created by the deposition of urate crystals (Fig. 15–1). Urate crystals are not radiographically opaque. However, calcium may precipitate with the urate crystals to varying degrees, creating variation in the density of tophi (Fig. 15–2). Tophi are usually found in the periarticular area along the extensor surface of bone. However, they may be intra-articular or not associated with the joint at all.

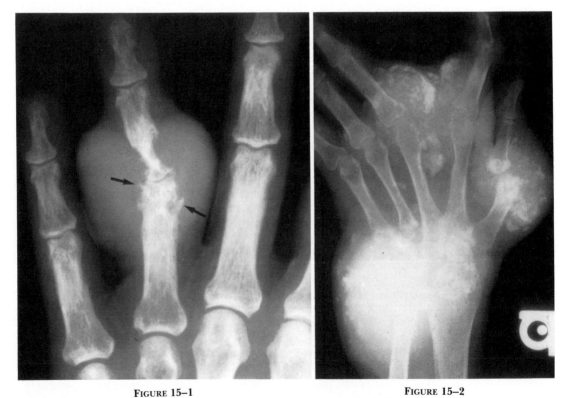

FIGURE 15–1   FIGURE 15–2

FIGURE 15–1. Gout involving the 4th digit. The soft tissue mass surrounding the PIP joint represents a tophus. Despite extensive involvement of the bone with erosion of the middle phalanx and bone spiculation (arrows) of the adjacent proximal phalanx, the PIP joint is only minimally narrowed. Mineralization is maintained.

FIGURE 15–2. AP view of the hand in severe tophaceous gout. Calcium has precipitated with the urate crystals, giving density to the tophi. (Courtesy of R. B. Harrison, University of Mississippi Medical Center, Jackson.)

Tophi over an extended period of time erode the underlying bone. Because of the indolence of the process, the erosion produced usually has a sclerotic border. The erosion looks "punched out" and has frequently been described as a "mouse bite" (Fig. 15–3). Often as the erosion is developing the proximal edge of cortex is remodeled in an outward direction, creating an overhanging edge (Fig. 15–4). This is seen in connection with 40 per cent of the erosions identified. If the tophus is intra-articular and involves adjacent bones, its extensor location and the indolence of the erosion allow preservation of the flexor portion of the joint space. Therefore on a radiograph, even when part of the joint is involved, the joint space appears to be preserved (Fig. 15–5). Urate crystals may deposit within the bone, producing an intraosseous tophus; the bone involved shows a lytic, expansile lesion with or without calcification (Fig.

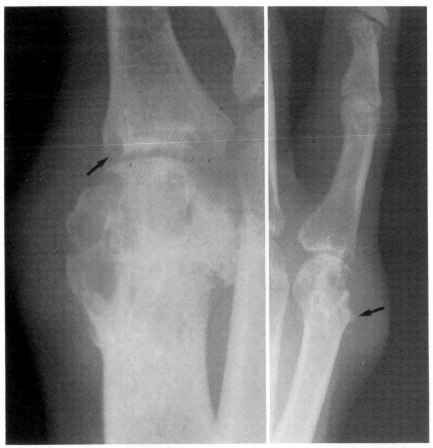

FIGURE 15–3   FIGURE 15–4

FIGURE 15–3. Erosive changes of gout in the 1st MTP joint. All erosions have sclerotic borders. One resembles a "mouse bite" (arrow).

FIGURE 15–4. Tophaceous gout involving the 5th MCP joint. A soft tissue tophus is present dorsally. The mineralization and joint space are maintained. The erosions have sclerotic borders. An overhanging edge of cortex is present (arrow). (From Brower AC: The radiologic approach to arthritis. Med Clin North Am 68:1593, 1984.)

15–6). Once the bone changes have occurred, they cannot be reversed; however, the urate crystals can disappear with treatment. Therefore it is possible to see the bone changes of chronic tophaceous gout without the presence of the actual tophi (Fig. 15–7).

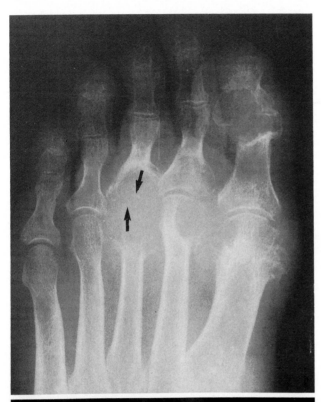

FIGURE 15–5. AP view of the foot with chronic tophaceous gout. Tophi involve the 1st, 2nd, and 3rd MTP joints and the 1st IP joint. Mineralization is maintained. Despite extensive erosion, the remaining joint space is preserved at each of the MTP joints. At the 3rd MTP joint only a ghost outline of the joint space is observed (arrows), showing preservation of the plantar aspect of the joint, which has not been eroded by the dorsal tophus.

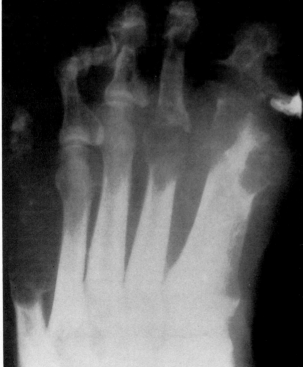

FIGURE 15–6. AP view of toes with tophaceous gout. The expansile lytic lesions involving the 5th proximal phalanx and metatarsal head and shaft represent intraosseous tophi.

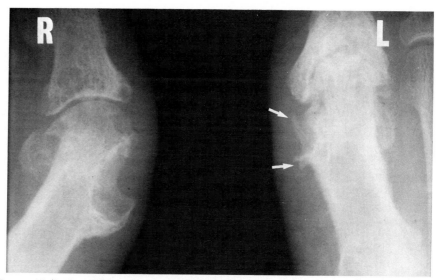

FIGURE 15–7. First MTP joints in treated gout. The large erosion with sclerotic border and overhanging edge of cortex involving the right metatarsal head was produced by a tophus that is no longer present. Urate crystals, no longer present, deposited in the soft tissues and the cartilage of the left MTP joint produced the joint space loss, the erosive changes, and the bone spiculation (arrow).

Normal mineralization is maintained. It is unusual to see even transient juxta-articular osteoporosis. Actually, bone production is a manifestation of the chronicity of the disease process. Bone production is seen as part of the osteoarthritic picture. It is also seen as the sclerotic border to the erosion and the overhanging edge of cortex. One may identify irregular bone spicules at sites of tendon and ligamentous attachment (Fig. 15–8). Enlargement of ends of bones may also occur.

The peripheral appendicular skeleton is the common site of involvement, with the foot being the classic location. It is extremely unusual to see the hip, shoulder, or spine involved with gout.

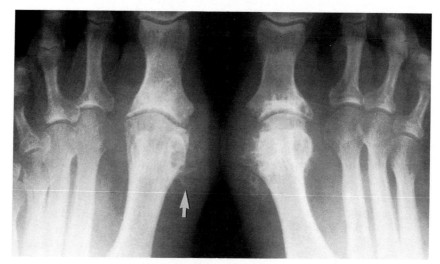

FIGURE 15–8. AP view of both metatarsal joints in long-standing gout. Bone spicules are present (arrow). Despite the erosions, the metatarsal heads appear enlarged.

THE FOOT

Sixty-five per cent of patients with gout experience their first attack in the 1st metatarsophalangeal joint (Figs. 15–7 to 15–9). Eventually, 90 per cent of patients with gout have involvement of this particular joint. Sometimes it is difficult to distinguish gout from osteoarthritis in this particular joint. Both may present with a hallux valgus deformity and productive bone changes. However, the tophus is usually present on the dorsal aspect of the joint and causes erosive changes on the dorsal surface of the 1st metatarsal head and to a lesser extent the adjacent proximal phalanx. In particular, the lateral view of the 1st MTP joint shows this tophus and erosion and distinguishes the process from the osteophytic and cystic changes of osteoarthritis (Fig. 15–10). The erosion may present medially on the 1st metatarsal head, and the tophus may be mistaken for a bunion (Fig. 15–11). Certainly presence of the overhanging edge of cortex distinguishes this from the cystic change of osteoarthritis. After the 1st MTP joint, the 1st IP joint and the 5th MTP joint are favored areas of involvement. However, any of the MTP joints may be involved (Fig. 15–5).

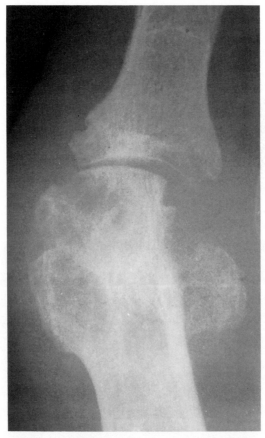

FIGURE 15–9. The first MTP joint in gout. The proximal phalanx is subluxed laterally in relationship to the metatarsal head. Erosions with sclerotic borders are present. The joint space is minimally narrowed.

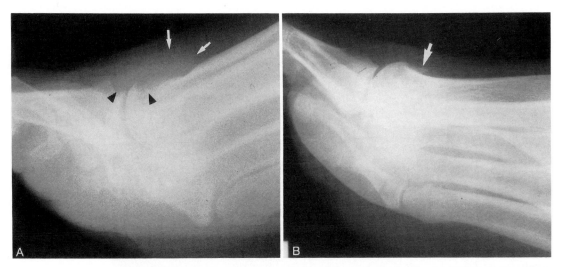

FIGURE 15–10. Gout versus osteoarthritis. *A,* Lateral view of the 1st MTP joint in gout. A tophus is present dorsal to the 1st MTP joint (arrows). Bone erosion is present dorsally (arrowheads). *B,* Lateral view of the 1st MTP joint in osteoarthritis. There is neither an identifiable tophus nor erosion. An osteophyte is present (arrow).

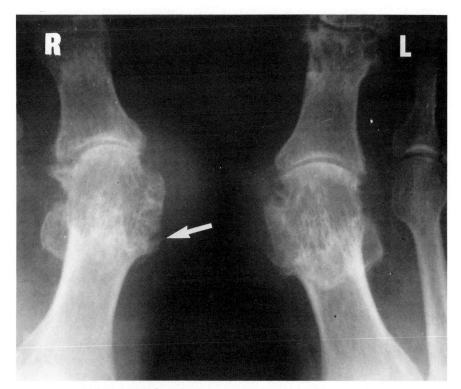

FIGURE 15–11. The first MTP joints in gout. While the osteophyte, subchondral sclerosis, and soft tissue mass at the right MTP joint might be interpreted as osteoarthritis with a bunion, the erosion with the overhanging edge of bone (arrow) indicates the correct diagnosis of gout. The changes in the left MTP joint are classic for gout.

The tarsal area is involved frequently, with swelling over the dorsum of the foot. Any of the tarsal joints may be involved (Fig. 15–12); however, there seems to be preference for the tarsometatarsal joints. Extensive destruction in this area by gout still produces punched-out erosions with sclerotic borders (Fig. 15–13).

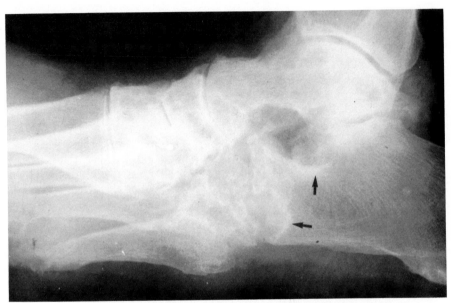

FIGURE 15–12. Lateral view of the foot in gout. Large erosions with sclerotic borders are seen in the calcaneus as it articulates with the cuboid and the talus (arrows).

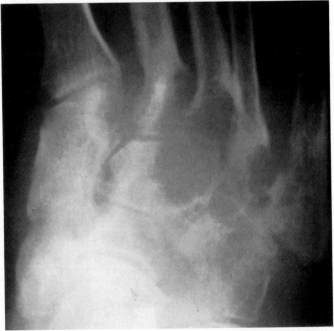

FIGURE 15–13. Midfoot in gout. There are extensive erosive changes involving the tarsometatarsal joint spaces.

THE HAND

The hand, like the foot, is involved in a sporadic asymmetrical fashion (Fig. 15–14). No one joint is preferred over another in the fingers. Mineralization is maintained. Tophi may or may not be identified. If erosive changes are present, erosive areas have sclerotic borders and perhaps overhanging edges of cortex. The joint space may or may not be preserved. One may see a sporadic atypical distribution of osteoarthritic changes. There may be pancarpal involvement of the wrist; however, frequently there is preferential involvement of the carpometacarpal joint space with erosive change (Fig. 15–15).

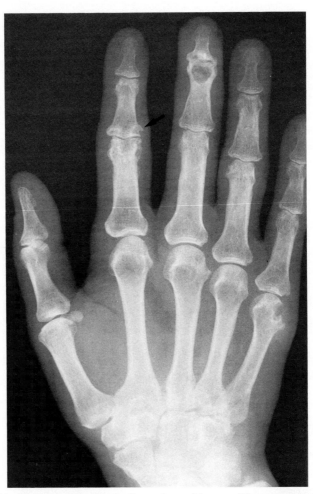

FIGURE 15–14. AP view of the hand of a patient with gout. Mineralization is normal. A tophus and associated erosion with a sclerotic border and overhanging edge of cortex are present at the 5th MCP joint. The 2nd PIP joint shows enlargement of the bone ends with osteophytes and osteoarthritic bone spicules (arrow). The 3rd DIP joint shows secondary osteoarthritic changes and an intraosseous tophus in the distal end of the middle phalanx. These changes represent the spectrum of gout.

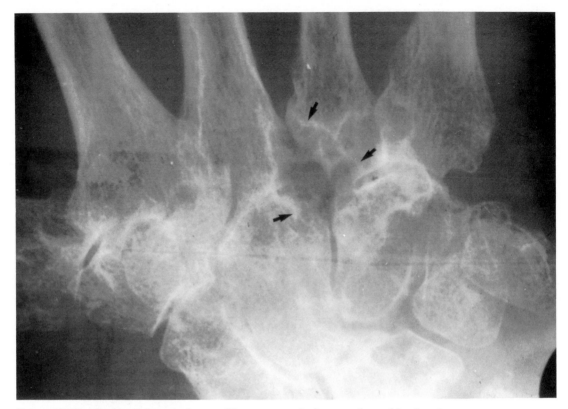

FIGURE 15–15. AP view of the wrist in gout. There are punched-out erosions with sclerotic borders involving the base of the 3rd, 4th, and 5th metacarpals as they articulate with the capitate and hamate (arrows).

THE ELBOW

The elbow is involved in 30 per cent of patients with gout. There is preferential olecranon bursal involvement with swelling over the extensor surface. Gout must always be considered in a patient with unilateral olecranon bursitis and is usually the diagnosis in a patient with bilateral olecranon bursitis (Fig. 15–16). The adjacent bone may or may not be involved. If it is involved, there may be either erosive (Fig. 15–17) or proliferative changes (Fig. 15–16) present.

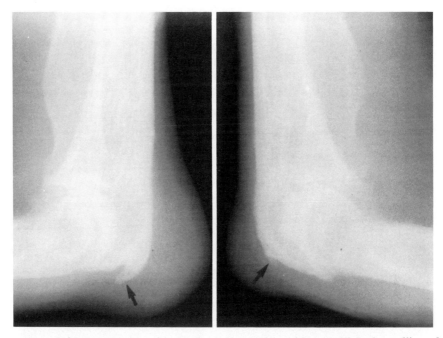

FIGURE 15–16. Lateral view of both elbows in a patient with gout. There is swelling of both olecranon bursae. There is also bone proliferation at both olecranons (arrows).

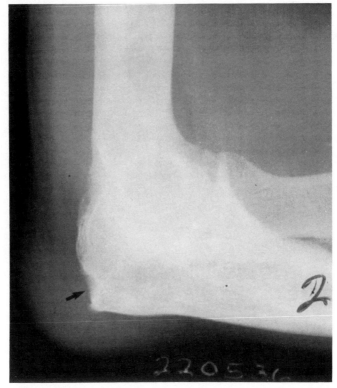

FIGURE 15–17. Lateral view of the elbow in gout. Bursitis is present. Erosion (arrow) is present in the olecranon.

OTHER APPENDICULAR SITES

The ankle and knee are frequently affected. The ankle tends to present the picture of tophaceous gout (Fig. 15–18), whereas the knee tends to present the picture of osteoarthritis. The hip and shoulder are rarely involved.

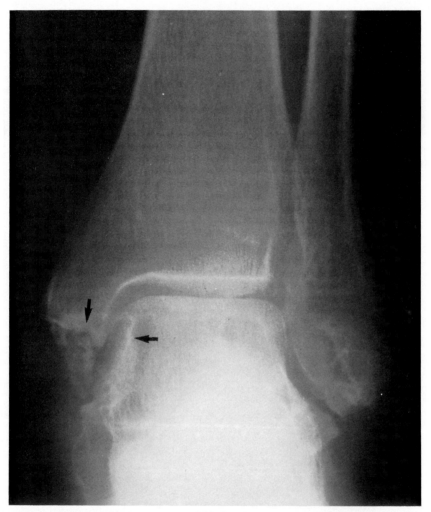

FIGURE 15–18. The ankle in gout. A calcified tophus is present inferior to the medial malleolus. Adjacent erosive changes with sclerotic borders are present (arrows).

THE SACROILIAC JOINT

Twelve per cent of the patients with radiographic gout have involvement of the sacroiliac joint. Five per cent present with an osteoarthritic picture indistinguishable from any secondary osteoarthritis. Seven per cent show a classic change in the synovial aspect of the sacroiliac joint. There is a huge punched-out erosion with a sclerotic border (Fig. 15–19). A bone spicule representing an overhanging edge of cortex may be present. These changes are produced by a tophus. The tophus itself may or may not be seen, depending upon the degree of calcification.

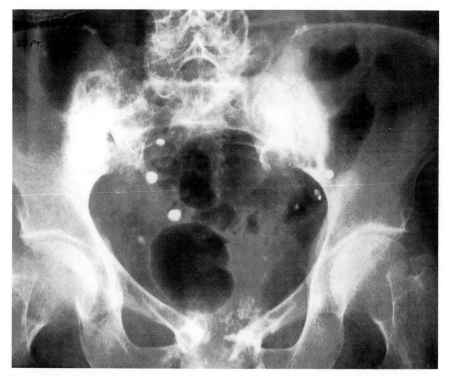

FIGURE 15–19. AP view of the pelvis in a patient with gout. Tophaceous deposits are present in the pubic symphysis and both sacroiliac joints. There are associated erosive changes with sclerotic borders and reparative bone.

SUMMARY

The radiographic changes of gout are identified relatively late in the disease process. The changes fit into two categories: (1) that of osteoarthritis indistinguishable from other causes of secondary osteoarthritis, and (2) changes that are pathognomonic of chronic tophaceous deposit.

SUGGESTED READINGS

Bloch C, Hermann G, Yu TF: A radiological re-evaluation of gout: A study of 2000 patients. AJR 134:781–787, 1980.

Martel W: Radiology of the rheumatic diseases. In Hollander JL, McCarty DJ Jr (eds.): Arthritis and Allied Conditions. 8th ed. Philadelphia, Lea & Febiger, 1972, p 115.

Martel W: The overhanging margin of bone: A roentgenologic manifestation of gout. Radiology 91:755, 1968.

Resnick D: The radiographic manifestations of gouty arthritis. CRC Crit Rev Diag Imaging 9:265–335, 1977.

Vyhnanek L, Lavick J, Blahos J: Roentgenological findings in gout. Radiol Clin 29:256, 1960.

Watt I, Middlemiss H: The radiology of gout. Clin Radiol 26:27, 1975.

Wright JT: Unusual manifestations of gout. Australas Radiol 10:365, 1966.

CALCIUM PYROPHOSPHATE DIHYDRATE (CPPD) CRYSTAL DEPOSITION DISEASE

Calcium pyrophosphate dihydrate (CPPD) crystal deposition disease is a common disorder and the most common crystal arthropathy. In a typical hospital population, one to three patients per week will be observed with some manifestation of this disorder. It typically affects the middle-aged and elderly population. Some estimate the frequency to be 5 per cent of this population. The clinical picture varies from the pseudogout syndrome to asymptomatic joint disease. The radiographic picture also varies from chondrocalcinosis without arthropathy to severe arthropathy.

Chondrocalcinosis is the deposition of CPPD crystals into fibrous and/ or hyaline cartilage. Chondrocalcinosis has been associated in the past with many diseases such as diabetes, degenerative joint disease, and gout. However, the only two diseases that have definite significant association with CPPD crystal deposition are primary hyperparathyroidism and hemochromatosis. If a patient with gout demonstrates chondrocalcinosis on the radiograph, the chondrocalcinosis is not secondary to deposition of urate crystals but secondary to deposition of CPPD crystals. The patient should be diagnosed as having two separate diseases, gout and CPPD crystal deposition disease (Fig. 16–1). In ochronosis, some patients have had CPPD crystals in the synovium but not in the cartilage.

Chondrocalcinosis is seen most frequently in the knee, pubic symphysis, and wrist (Fig. 16–2). At least one of these areas is involved in a patient with CPPD deposition disease. Therefore, when screening a patient for this disorder, one should obtain radiographs of these areas. Radiographic diagnosis can be made when two or more areas in the skeleton demonstrate chondrocalcinosis. CPPD crystals may also deposit in synovium capsules, tendons, and ligaments.

The arthropathy of CPPD radiographically resembles osteoarthritis. However, its distribution within the skeleton as well as within the individual joint is distinctive, allowing separation from primary or mechanical osteoarthritis. The radiographic features of CPPD crystal deposition disease are the following:

1. **Chondrocalcinosis**

2. **Normal mineralization**

3. **Uniform joint space loss**

4. **Subchondral new bone formation**

5. **Variable osteophyte formation**

6. **Cysts—more prominent than in osteoarthritis**

7. **Occasional neuropathic changes**

8. **Bilateral distribution**

9. **Distribution in knees, hands, and hips in decreasing order of frequency; unlike osteoarthritis, the shoulder and elbow are involved.**

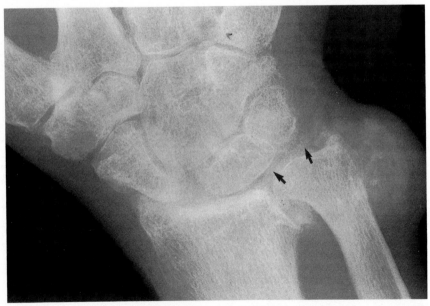

FIGURE 16–1. The wrist in a patient with gout and CPPD crystal deposition disease. The calcified mass lateral to the distal ulna is a calcified tophus of gout. Chondrocalcinosis (arrows) is also present, indicating CPPD crystal deposition disease.

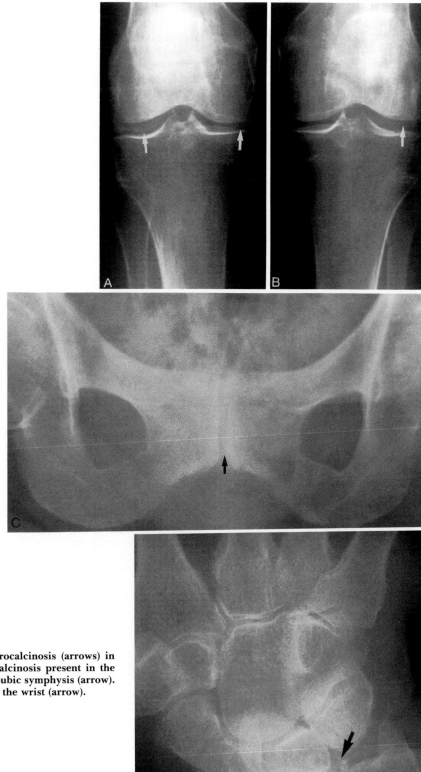

FIGURE 16–2. *A*, Chondrocalcinosis (arrows) in the knees. *B*, Chondrocalcinosis present in the fibrous cartilage of the pubic symphysis (arrow). *C*, Chondrocalcinosis in the wrist (arrow).

THE KNEE

The knee is the most commonly involved joint in CPPD crystal deposition disease. Eighty per cent show chondrocalcinosis, and 75 per cent show changes of an arthropathy. The chondrocalcinosis is seen as (1) wedge-shaped calcification in the fibrocartilaginous menisci and (2) thin linear calcification in hyaline cartilage paralleling the femoral condyles or tibial plateau (Fig. 16–3). Calcification may also be seen in the synovium, quadriceps tendon, or cruciate ligaments.

In the arthropathy there is often preferential narrowing of the patellofemoral joint space with sparing of the medial and lateral tibiofemoral compartments (Fig. 16–3). This patellofemoral narrowing is accompanied by subchondral bone sclerosis and osteophyte formation on the posterior aspect of the patella and the anterior aspect of the femoral condyles. There is often a scalloped defect seen in the femur proximal to the patella in the flexed knee. This scalloping is caused by abutment of the patella against the femur when the knee is in extension. Isolated patellofemoral involvement in the knee should always suggest CPPD crystal deposition disease.

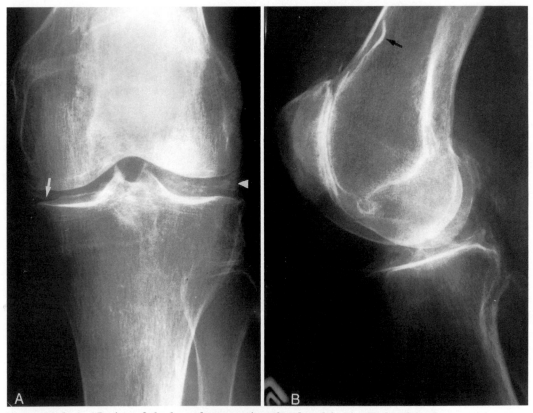

FIGURE 16–3. *A*, AP view of the knee demonstrating chondrocalcinosis. Wedge-shaped calcification is seen in the fibrocartilaginous meniscus (arrowhead), and curvilinear calcification is seen in the hyaline cartilage (arrow). The medial and lateral tibiofemoral joint spaces are preserved. *B*, Lateral view of the knee. There is total loss of the patellofemoral joint space with subchondral sclerosis and osteophyte formation. There is a scalloped defect (arrow) where the patella abuts the femur in extension. (*B* From Brower AC: The radiologic approach to arthritis. Med Clin North Am 68:1593, 1984.)

However, the other compartments in the knee may become involved, with the medial tibiofemoral compartment being involved more frequently than the lateral tibiofemoral compartment. In this case, the presence of chondrocalcinosis may be the only finding to distinguish this arthropathy from mechanical osteoarthritis. Occasionally the osteoarthritic changes become so severe as to resemble a neuropathic joint (Fig. 16–4). Such excessive changes should suggest CPPD arthropathy, rather than mechanical osteoarthritis.

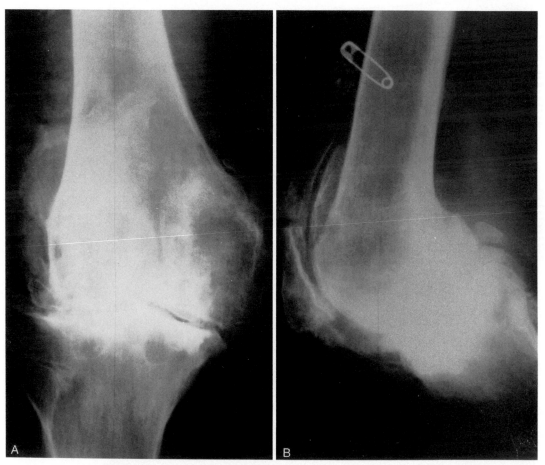

FIGURE 16–4. AP (*A*) and lateral (*B*) views of a knee in CPPD arthropathy. There is loss of all compartments of the knee joint. There is extensive subchondral sclerosis and some cyst formation. There is fragmentation and bone debris in the joint. The findings resemble those of a neuropathic joint.

THE HAND

Chondrocalcinosis in the wrist is found in 65 per cent of the patients and the arthropathy in 70 per cent of the patients. Chondrocalcinosis is most frequently seen in the triangular fibrocartilage (Fig. 16–5). The hyaline cartilage may calcify around any of the carpal bones but most frequently between the navicular and lunate. This may lead to disruption of a ligament between the navicular and lunate with subsequent separation or dissociation of the two bones. In the fingers pyrophosphate deposition tends to occur in the synovium and capsule around the MCP joints (Fig. 16–6).

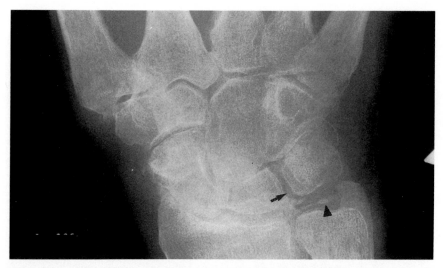

FIGURE 16–5. The wrist in CPPD arthropathy. There is chondrocalcinosis present in the triangular fibrocartilage (arrowhead) and in the hyaline cartilage between the lunate and triquetrium (arrow). There is also loss of the joint space between the navicular and the radius and between the lunate and capitate with subchondral bone formation.

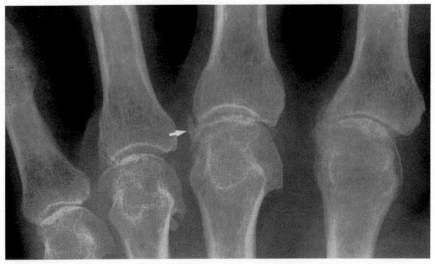

FIGURE 16–6. MCP joints in CPPD arthropathy. Calcification is present in the capsule (arrow). There is loss of joint space, osteophyte formation, and subchondral sclerosis.

The arthropathy in the hands is usually confined to the MCP joints. The IP joints are usually spared. The changes are those of osteoarthritis in the wrong distribution for primary osteoarthritis. There is joint space narrowing, subchondral bone formation, and variable osteophyte formation (Fig. 16–7). Occasionally there is cyst formation and resultant bone collapse. The arthropathy of the wrist most commonly affects the radiocarpal joint. Again, there are osteoarthritic changes in a distribution different from that of primary osteoarthritis. There is joint space narrowing, subchondral bone formation, and cyst formation (Fig. 16–8). The later may dominate the radiographic picture. If there is dissociation between the navicular and lunate, there may be accompanying narrowing of the joint space between the lunate and capitate. The appearance has been described as a "stepladder" configuration (Fig. 16–9).

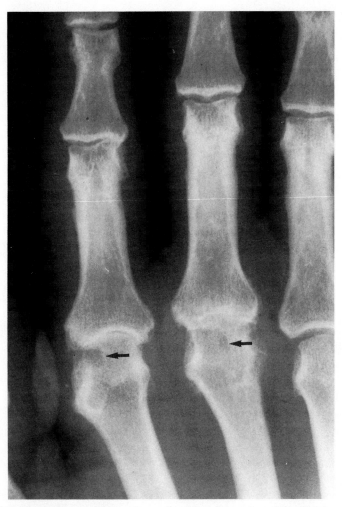

FIGURE 16–7. Two digits in CPPD arthropathy. There is sparing of the IP joints. There is loss of the MCP joints with osteophyte formation and subchondral sclerosis. There is also cyst formation present (arrows).

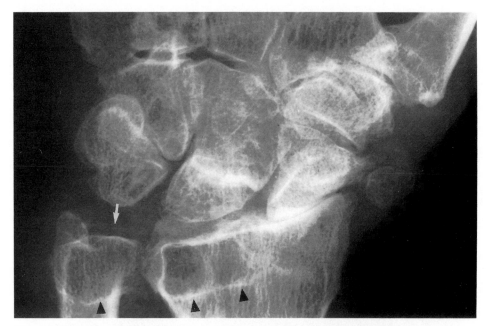

FIGURE 16–8. A wrist with CPPD arthropathy. Chondrocalcinosis is present (arrow). Osteoarthritic changes are present involving the radiocarpal joint and the lunate-capitate joint. Large cysts are present in the distal ulna and radius (arrowheads).

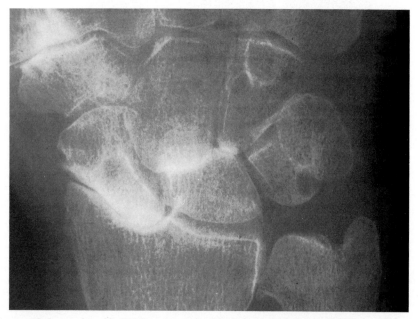

FIGURE 16–9. A wrist with CPPD arthropathy. There is total loss of the joint space between the navicular and the radius as well as the capitate and lunate with subchondral sclerosis. This is the classic "step-ladder" configuration. (Courtesy of Dr. C. S. Resnik, University of Maryland.)

THE HIP

Chondrocalcinosis is present in the hip in 45 per cent of patients and the arthropathy in 30 per cent of patients with CPPD. Chondrocalcinosis is seen as calcification of the fibrocartilage of the acetabular labrum and calcification of the hyaline cartilage paralleling the femoral head (Fig. 16–10). Most commonly the arthropathy causes uniform loss of cartilage and resultant axial migration of the femoral head within the acetabulum. This cartilage loss is accompanied by osteoarthritic changes (Fig. 16–11). However, the osteophytes may not be as large as those seen in osteoarthritis, and subchondral cyst formation may dominate the picture (Fig. 16–12). If the axis of weight bearing remains in its normal position, there is absence of the huge medial osteophyte and new bone apposition along the medial cortex of the femoral neck so commonly identified with osteoarthritis. Occasionally there may be bone collapse, destruction, and fragmentation leading to the appearance of a neuropathic joint.

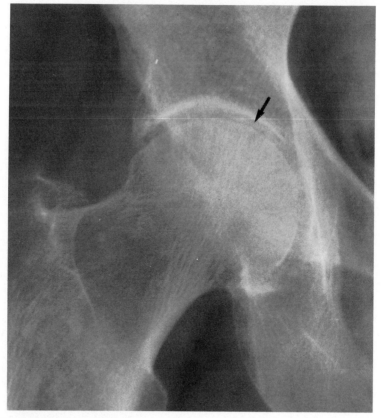

FIGURE 16–10. AP view of the hip demonstrating presence of chondrocalcinosis (arrow) without associated arthropathy.

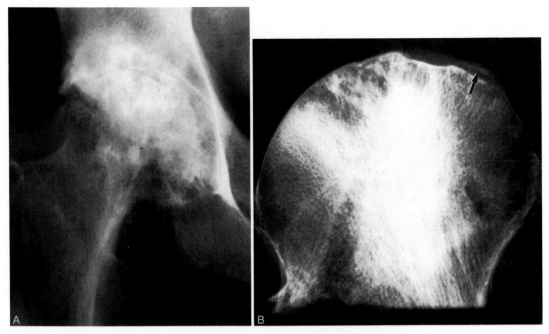

FIGURE 16–11. *A*, AP view of the hip with CPPD arthropathy. There is uniform loss of the cartilage with axial migration of the femoral head within the acetabulum. There are subchondral sclerosis and osteophyte formation present. *B*, Specimen radiograph of the same femoral head. The arrow points to chondrocalcinosis of the hyaline cartilage which was not visible on the routine radiograph.

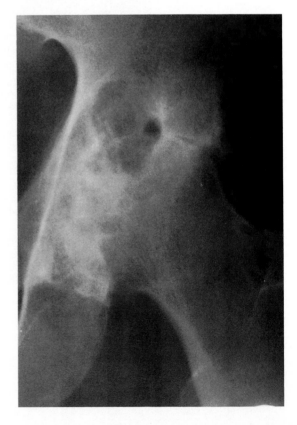

FIGURE 16–12. AP view of a hip with CPPD arthropathy. There is uniform cartilage loss with axial migration of the femoral head within the acetabulum. There are subchondral sclerosis and extensive subchondral cyst formation. There is relative absence of osteophyte formation. There is no evidence of new bone apposition along the femoral neck. (From Brower AC: The radiologic approach to arthritis. Med Clin North Am 68:1593, 1984.)

OTHER APPENDICULAR SITES

Unlike primary osteoarthritis, the non–weight-bearing joints, or the elbow and shoulder, are frequently involved. Again, chondrocalcinosis is seen more commonly than the actual arthropathy (Fig. 16–13). In both these areas, the arthropathy is one of osteoarthritis with subchondral bone formation, osteophyte formation, and subchondral cyst formation (Fig.16–14). Similar changes may be seen in the acromioclavicular joint. The foot and ankle are less frequently involved. Chondrocalcinosis may be identified anywhere. Calcification may be seen in the synovium and capsule around the metatarsophalangeal joints. In the foot, the arthropathy has a predilection for the talonavicular joint.

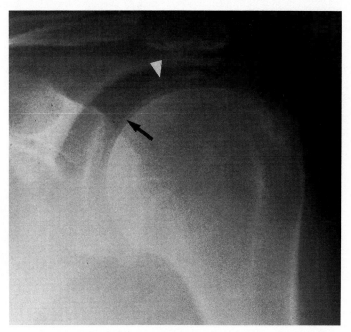

FIGURE 16–13. AP view of the shoulder demonstrating chondrocalcinosis of the hyaline cartilage (arrow) and CPPD crystal deposition in adjacent soft tissue structures (arrowhead).

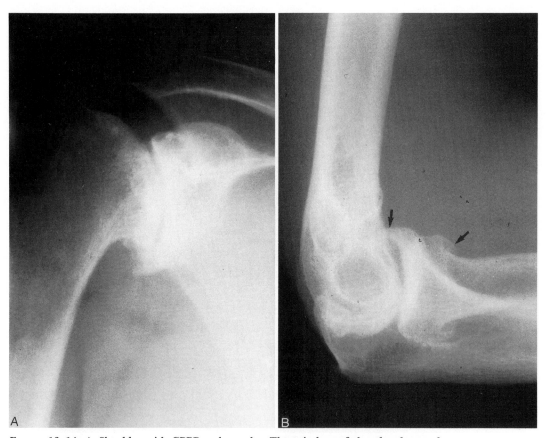

FIGURE 16–14. *A*, Shoulder with CPPD arthropathy. There is loss of the glenohumeral joint space with subchondral sclerosis, osteophyte formation, and subchondral cyst formation. *B*, Elbow with CPPD arthropathy. There is loss of the joint space with subchondral sclerosis and osteophyte formation (arrows).

THE SPINE

Spinal involvement is not uncommon and should be considered in any patient with evidence of degenerative disc disease at multiple levels. There is an increased incidence of the vacuum phenomenon at more than one level (Fig. 16–15). The diagnosis can be further defined by observing calcification in the soft tissue structures around the intervertebral disc space. The apophyseal joints may be involved as well, with osteoarthritic changes and resultant spondylolisthesis.

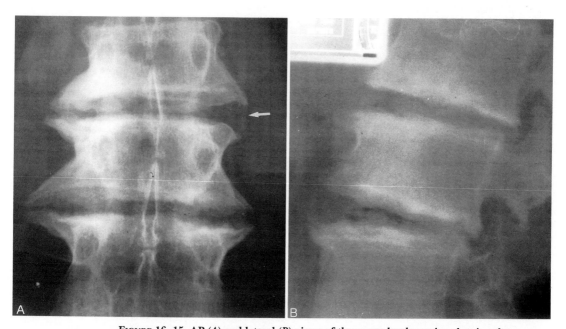

FIGURE 16–15. AP (A) and lateral (B) views of the upper lumbar spine showing the vacuum phenomenon at two disc levels. There is adjacent subchondral sclerosis and osteophyte formation. There is also calcification present in the soft tissue structures at the level of the disc (arrow).

SUMMARY

The radiographic hallmarks of CPPD crystal deposition disease are chondrocalcinosis and osteoarthritic changes in a specific distribution. Even in the absence of chondrocalcinosis the specific distribution of osteoarthritic changes should suggest the correct diagnosis.

SUGGESTED READINGS

Lagier R: Femoral cortical erosions and osteoarthrosis of the knee with chondrocalcinosis. An anatomo-radiological study of two cases. Fortschr Geb Roentgenstr Nuklearmed 120:460–467, 1974.

Martel W, Champion CK, Thompson GR, et al.: A roentgenologically distinctive arthropathy in some patients with the pseudogout syndrome. AJR 109:587–605, 1970.

Martel W, McCarter DK, Solsky MA, et al.: Further observations on the arthropathy of calcium pyrophosphate crystal deposition disease. Radiology 141:1–15, 1981.

McCarty DJ Jr: Calcium pyrophosphate dihydrate crystal deposition disease—1975. Arthritis Rheum 19(Suppl):275–285, 1976.

Resnick D, Niwayama G: Calcium pyrophosphate dihydrate (CPPD) crystal deposition disease. In Resnick D, Niwayama G (eds.): Diagnosis of Bone and Joint Disorders. Philadelphia, W.B. Saunders Company, 1981, p 1520.

Resnick D, Niwayama G, Goergen TG, et al.: Clinical, radiographic and pathologic abnormalities in calcium pyrophosphate dihydrate deposition disease (CPPD): Pseudogout. Radiology 122:1–15, 1977.

Resnik CS, Miller BW, Gelberman RH, et al.: Hand and wrist involvement in calcium pyrophosphate dihydrate crystal deposition disease. J Hand Surg 8:856, 1983.

Resnik CS, Resnick D: Calcium pyrophosphate dihydrate crystal deposition disease. Curr Probl Diagn Radiol 11(6):1–40, 1982.

Zitnan D, Sitaj S: Natural course of articular chondrocalcinosis. Arthritis Rheum 19(Suppl):363, 1976.

chapter 17

HYDROXYAPATITE DEPOSITION DISEASE (HADD)

Hydroxyapatite deposition disease (HADD) is an extremely common disorder causing periarticular disease in the form of tendinitis or bursitis. Only rarely does it cause true articular disease. Calcium hydroxyapatite deposits in muscles, capsules, bursae, and tendon sheaths. Although this deposition is associated with many systemic diseases, such as collagen vascular diseases, renal osteodystrophy, hypervitaminosis D, and milk-alkali syndrome, in many patients it occurs idiopathically with no underlying systemic problem. The radiographic findings are the following:

1. Periarticular calcification
    A. Early deposition is linear and poorly defined, often blending with the soft tissues
    B. With time this calcification becomes denser, homogeneous, well delineated, and circular

2. Soft tissue swelling

3. Normal adjacent joint and bone

4. Occasional joint effusion

5. Occasional osteoporosis; occasional reactive sclerosis

6. Single joint distribution. Occasionally multiple joints may be involved either at the same time (33 per cent) or successively (67 per cent).

7. Distribution in shoulder, hip, wrist, elbow, and neck in decreasing order of frequency

SHOULDER

The shoulder is the most common site of calcific tendinitis or bursitis. Calcium hydroxyapatite is said to be observed in 40 per cent of the shoulders radiographed for shoulder pain. It usually locates first in a tendon. The actual tendon location can be identified by changes in rotation of the humerus on the radiograph (Fig. 17–1). Fifty-two per cent of the calcific tendinitis occurs in the supraspinatus tendon, which can be seen in profile over the greater tuberosity on external rotation. Calcification in the infraspinatus tendon profiles laterally on internal rotation. Calcification of the teres minor also profiles laterally on internal rotation, but is inferior to the infraspinatus calcification. Calcification in the subscapularis profiles medially on internal rotation. Calcification of the long head of the biceps is seen on the superior aspect of the glenoid; that of the short head of the biceps is seen on the tip of the coracoid. Rotation does not change the location of calcification in the biceps.

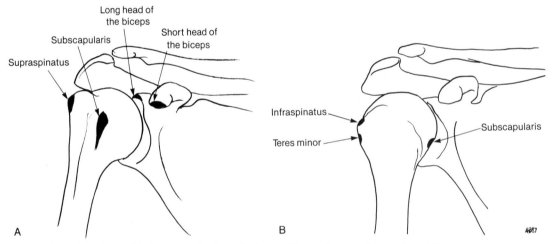

FIGURE 17–1. Locations of hydroxyapatite deposits in specific tendons as observed on AP view of the shoulder in (A) external rotation and (B) internal rotation.

Calcification in the rotator cuff area may eventually rupture into the bursa (Fig. 17–2). In some patients this has led to a secondary severe destructive arthropathy. The result of this particular sequence of events has been labeled the "Milwaukee" shoulder.

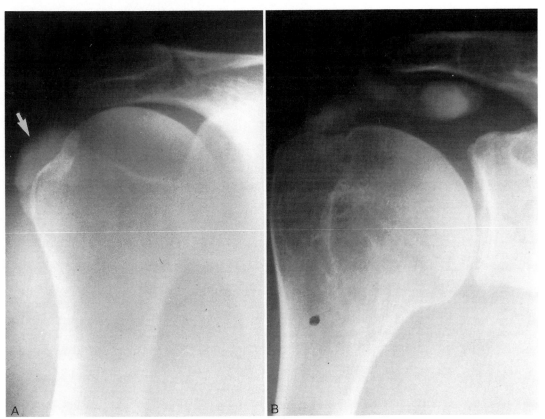

FIGURE 17–2. *A*, AP view of the shoulder showing a large amorphous calcific deposit in the area of the rotator cuff attachment (arrow). *B*, AP view of the same shoulder demonstrating amorphous calcification not only in the rotator cuff attachment but also in the subacromial bursa.

OTHER SITES

Around the hip hydroxyapatite deposition may occur in the gluteal insertions into the greater trochanter and surrounding bursa. These calcifications may appear linear or cloud-like (Fig. 17–3). Calcification in the elbow occurs around the medial and lateral condyles of the humerus or in the triceps as it inserts into the olecranon (Fig. 17–4).

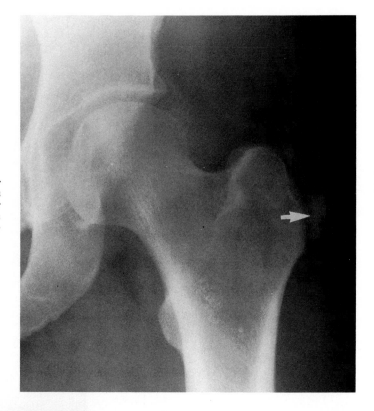

FIGURE 17–3. AP view of the hip demonstrating hydroxyapatite deposition into the gluteal insertions at the greater trochanter (arrow). The calcifications are both cloud-like and linear in their appearance.

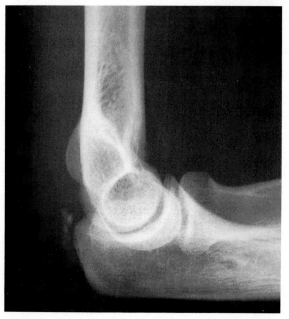

FIGURE 17–4. Lateral view of the elbow demonstrating calcification in the triceps as it inserts into the olecranon.

In the wrist the most frequent deposition occurs in the flexor carpi ulnaris. This is observed as calcification adjacent to the pisiform. Calcification may also be seen volar to the radiocarpal joint in the flexor carpi radialis, or adjacent to the distal ulna and ulna styloid in the extensor carpi ulnaris (Fig. 17–5). Tendinitis may cause adjacent bone osteoporosis (Fig. 17–6).

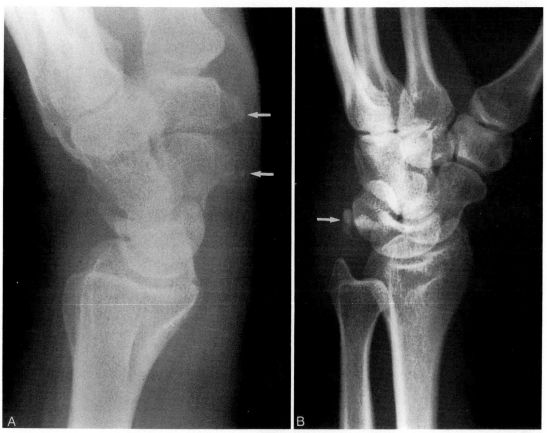

FIGURE 17–5. *A*, Lateral view of the wrist demonstrating calcification volar to the navicular and greater multangular (arrows), most likely in the flexor carpi radialis. *B*, Oblique view of the wrist demonstrating calcification adjacent to the triquetrium and distal to the ulna (arrow). This most likely is in the extensor carpi ulnaris.

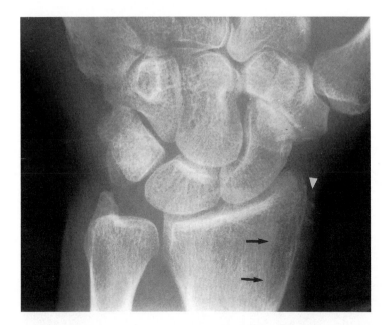

FIGURE 17–6. PA view of the wrist showing calcification in the soft tissue radial to the radial styloid (arrowhead). The bone adjacent to this calcification is reacting with osteoporosis (arrows).

Perhaps the most painful hydroxyapatite deposition occurs in the neck in the longus colli muscle, which is the chief flexor of the cervical spine. The patient usually complains of tremendous pain on swallowing. Radiographically, one observes soft tissue swelling and amorphous calcification anterior to the C2 vertebral body just inferior to the body of the atlas (Fig. 17–7).

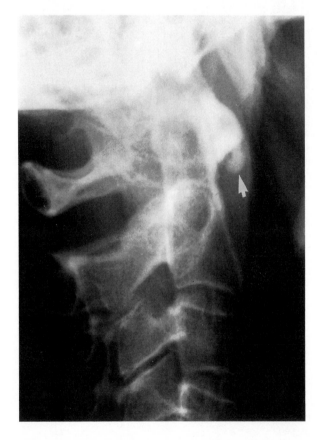

FIGURE 17–7. Lateral view of the upper cervical spine showing amorphous calcification inferior to the atlas and anterior to C2 lying in the longus colli muscle (arrow). There is adjacent soft tissue swelling.

It is now recognized that hydroxyapatite can deposit intra-articularly. Both periarticular and intra-articular deposition can lead to an arthropathy (Fig. 17–8). Most of the time an osteoarthritic radiographic picture has been described as part of the arthropathy. However, a severely destructive arthropathy has also been described involving the hand as well as the shoulder.

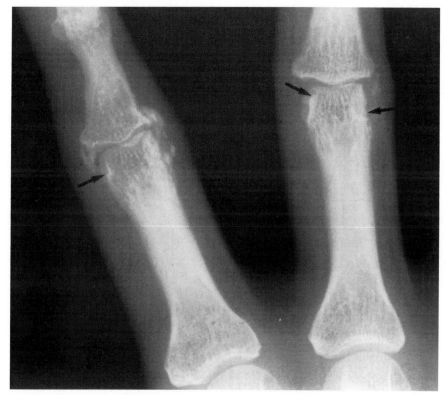

FIGURE 17–8. Two digits showing intra- and periarticular deposition of hydroxyapatite crystals. There is loss of the joint space as well as erosive changes (arrows).

SUMMARY

Hydroxyapatite deposition disease (HADD) is an extremely common disorder causing periarticular disease and only rarely intra-articular disease. The diagnosis is easily made by identifying calcification in the appropriate location. One must be careful to exclude an underlying systemic disease as the cause of this deposition.

SUGGESTED READINGS

Bonavita JA, Dalinka MK, Schumacher HR Jr: Hydroxyapatite deposition disease. Radiology 134:621–625, 1980.

Dalinka MK, Stewart V, Bomalaski JS, et al.: Periarticular calcifications in association with intra-articular corticosteroid injections (IACI). Radiology 153:615, 1984.

Dieppe PA, Huskisson EC, Crocker P, et al.: Apatite deposition disease: A new arthropathy. Lancet 1:266–269, 1976.

Haun CL: Retropharyngeal tendinitis. AJR 130:1137–1140, 1978.

McCarty DJ, Halverson PB, Carrera GR, et al.: "Milwaukee shoulder"—association of microspheroids containing hydroxyapatite crystals, active collagenase, and neutral protease with rotator cuff defects. I. Clinical aspects. Arthritis Rheum 24:464–472, 1981.

Pinals RS, Short CL: Calcific periarthritis involving multiple sites. Arthritis Rheum 9:566–574, 1966.

Schumacher HR, Miller JL, Ludivico C, Jessar RA: Erosive arthritis associated with apatite crystal deposition. Arthritis Rheum 24:31–37, 1981.

chapter 18

MISCELLANEOUS DEPOSITION DISEASES

Three deposition diseases are discussed in this chapter, all of which are extremely rare. All have been associated with radiographic chondrocalcinosis, or calcification of hyaline or fibrous cartilage. However, if chondrocalcinosis is defined as the deposition of calcium pyrophosphate dihydrate crystals into hyaline or fibrous cartilage, its association with all of these diseases becomes questionable. Whatever substance is deposited into the cartilage, degeneration and secondary osteoarthritis occur. Each of these diseases has specific changes that distinguish it from other arthropathies.

HEMOCHROMATOSIS

Hemochromatosis is a rare inherited disorder that leads to massive iron deposition throughout the body. It leads to an arthropathy in 24 to 50 per cent of affected patients. The arthropathy may or may not have associated radiographic chondrocalcinosis. This raises some question about the cause of the arthropathy. Although chondrocalcinosis is frequently observed, it has not been determined whether the calcium pyrophosphate dihydrate (CPPD) crystals actually cause degeneration of the cartilage or the crystals are deposited secondarily in already degenerated cartilage. It is known that iron inhibits pyrophosphatase activity in the cartilage, leading to the precipitation of CPPD crystals; however, it is not known whether the iron or the CPPD crystals cause the initial degeneration of the cartilage.

The arthropathy of hemochromatosis is almost identical to that of CPPD crystal deposition in that the radiographic picture is one of osteoarthritis in atypical sites for primary osteoarthritis. As in pyrophosphate arthropathy, subchondral cysts dominate the picture, and uniform, rather than non-uniform, loss of joint space is the rule. However, there are subtle differences that distinguish hemochromatosis from CPPD arthropathy. The radiographic findings in hemochromatosis arthropathy are the following:

1. Osteoporosis

2. Chondrocalcinosis—there appears to be more hyaline cartilage calcification than fibrous cartilage calcification when compared to CPPD arthropathy

3. Uniform joint space loss

4. Subchondral sclerosis

5. Subchondral cyst formation

6. Beak-like osteophytes

7. Slow progression of disease—no excessive neuropathic changes as seen in CPPD

8. Bilateral symmetrical distribution

9. Distribution in hand and wrist initially and most frequently; late widespread involvement throughout the skeleton

The subtle changes that may distinguish hemochomatosis arthropathy from CPPD arthropathy are best seen in the hand and wrist.

Hand and Wrist

In the hand there is specific preference for the 2nd and 3rd MCP joints with or without involvement of the other MCP's and wrist (Fig. 18–1). There will be uniform loss of the joint space with subchondral sclerosis present. Small (1 to 3 mm) subchondral cysts may be identified. There is a characteristic osteophytic beak on the medial aspect of the 2nd and 3rd metacarpals. There may be flattening or collapse of the heads of the metacarpals (Fig. 18–2). The 4th and 5th MCP joints may be involved, but the IP joints are usually spared.

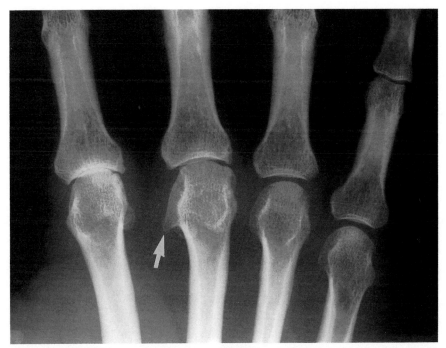

FIGURE 18–1. PA view of the 2nd through 5th MCP joints of a hand with hemochromatosis. The 4th and 5th MCP joints are not affected. The 2nd and 3rd MCP joints show marked loss of the joint space. A characteristic osteophytic beak is present on the medial aspect of the head of the 3rd metacarpal (arrow). There is flattening of both metacarpal heads.

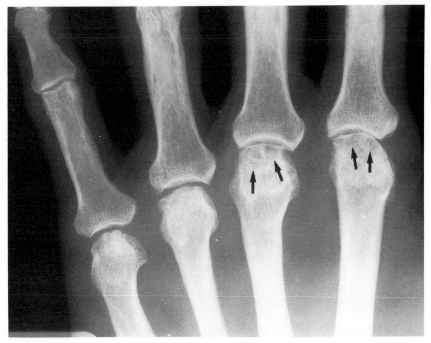

FIGURE 18–2. PA view of the MCP joints in a patient with hemochromatosis. In this case all of the MCP joints are involved. There is flattening of the metacarpal heads best illustrated in the 4th metacarpal head. There are numerous subchondral cysts present (arrows).

The distribution of the disease in the wrist differs from that in CPPD arthropathy. Although it may show preferential involvement for the radiocarpal compartment (Fig. 18–3) and the joint space between the capitate and lunate, as seen in CPPD arthropathy, it may involve primarily the common carpometacarpal and mid-carpal compartments, with sparing of the radiocarpal compartment. The changes seen are those of osteoarthritis in this distribution, with subchondral sclerosis and cyst formation.

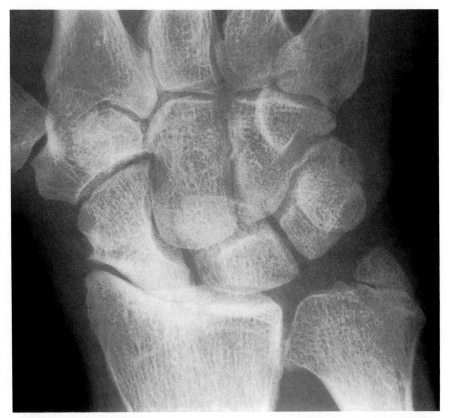

FIGURE 18–3. PA view of the wrist. There is loss of the radiocarpal joint space with secondary osteoarthritic changes. There is no evidence of chondrocalcinosis.

Other Joints

In some patients in the late phase of the disease there may be widespread involvement throughout the skeleton. It may be difficult to distinguish this involvement from that of CPPD arthropathy (Fig. 18–4). However, osteophytes, which have been described as "beak-like," may dominate the radiographic picture more frequently than in CPPD arthropathy. Generally the progression of the disease is very slow, whereas that in CPPD arthropathy can be extremely rapid. The kind of neuropathic changes seen in CPPD arthropathy are not seen in hemochromatosis.

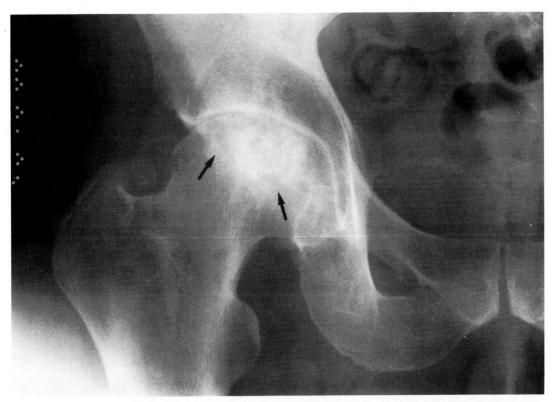

FIGURE 18–4. An AP view of the hip in a patient with hemochromatosis. There is axial migration of the femoral head within the acetabulum. There is extensive subchondral cyst formation more prominent in the femoral head (arrows). There is some reparative bone present. There is not extensive osteophytosis present. This appearance resembles that of CPPD arthropathy of the hip.

WILSON'S DISEASE

Wilson's disease is an extremely rare disease causing hepatolenticular degeneration. Copper is the substance deposited in the various tissues. The copper interferes with normal bone formation and causes osteopenic osteomalacia. An arthropathy occurs in 50 per cent of affected patients. However, the arthropathy is usually a radiographic finding rather than a clinical problem.

Radiographic chondrocalcinosis has been reported very rarely in this already rare disease. However, there is some question about the etiology of the cartilage calcification. Pathological proof of calcium pyrophosphate dihydrate crystal deposition has not been made. In vitro studies have shown that copper ions inhibit pyrophosphatase activity in cartilage, allowing pyrophosphate dihydrate crystal deposition, but this phenomenon has yet to be proven in vivo. There is considerable bone fragmentation in the joint in Wilson's disease, which could easily be mistaken for chondrocalcinosis.

The arthropathy of Wilson's disease is quite distinctive, with marked irregularity to the cortical and subchondral areas of the articular surface giving a "paint brush" appearance. There is significant subchondral bone fragmentation, which in larger joints may resemble osteochondritis dissecans. Well-corticated ossicles may be seen in the joint. Other than these specific changes, the arthropathy resembles an osteoarthritis in an unusual distribution for primary osteoarthritis. The arthropathy has been seen in the hand, wrist, foot, hip shoulder, elbow, and knee.

OCHRONOSIS

Ochronosis is perhaps the oldest known metabolic disease. Patients exhibit an absence of the enzyme homogentisic acid oxidase. This absence allows the accumulation of homogentisic acid, which deposits in collagen as a dark pigment. This ochronotic pigment is believed to be a polymer of homogentisic acid. When deposited in cartilage, it causes discoloration and then eventual fragmentation of the cartilage. Ochronotic pigment is not radiodense. The calcification observed in this disease is calcium hydroxyapatite.

The arthropathy of ochronosis is not usually identified until the fourth decade. Although it is a rare arthropathy, it is radiographically distinctive. The radiographic findings are the following:

1. Osteoporosis—diffuse

2. Disc degeneration at multiple levels, with calcification or a vacuum phenomenon present

3. Uniform joint space loss

4. Extensive subchondral sclerosis

5. Relative absence of osteophytes

6. Intra-articular loose bodies

7. Bilateral symmetrical distribution

8. Distribution in spine, knee, hip, and shoulder in decreasing order of frequency

The radiographic changes divide into spinal and extraspinal manifestations. The radiographic changes in the spine have been confused with ankylosing spondylitis; those outside the spine have been confused with primary osteoarthritis or CPPD crystal deposition disease. Careful observation of the radiographic changes will prevent these errors from being made.

The Spine

The lumbar spine is the site most frequently involved and the cervical spine the least frequently involved. Ochronotic pigment deposits in the disc, causing degeneration of the disc. This disc degeneration is present at multiple levels and is manifested radiographically as loss of disc height and presence of disc calcification and/or the vacuum phenomenon (Fig. 18–5). The calcification seen in the disc space is not the ochronotic pigment, but calcium hydroxyapatite, as seen in any degenerative disc disease. With progressive degeneration of the disc, the actual disc space may become totally obscured. Ossification of the discs has been noted in some instances with formation of very thick syndesmophytes between the vertebral bodies. Thus, the spine becomes ankylosed (Fig. 18–6).

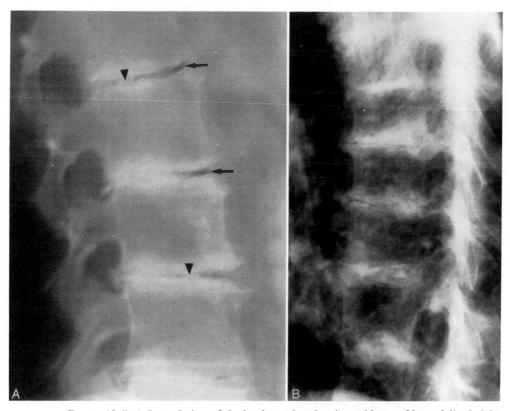

FIGURE 18–5. *A*, Lateral view of the lumbar spine showing evidence of loss of disc height at multiple levels. A vacuum phenomenon (arrows) and/or calcification (arrowheads) are seen at multiple levels. The bones are generally osteoporotic. The osteophytes are small and insignificant. *B*, Lateral view of the thoracic spine in ochronosis. The spine is generally osteoporotic. There is loss of disc height at all levels. There is disc calcification at all levels. There is a relative lack of osteophyte formation.

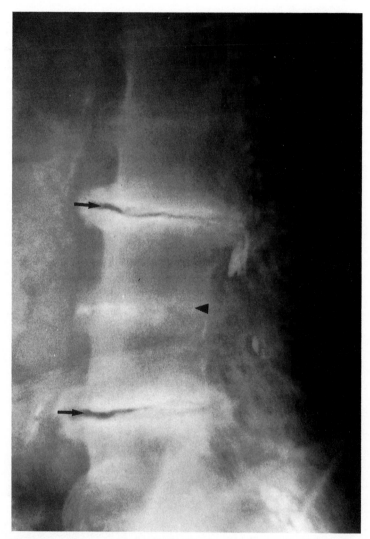

FIGURE 18–6. Lateral view of the lumbosacral spine in ochronosis. All disc spaces have been obliterated. A vacuum phenomenon is present at L2-L3 and L4-L5 (arrows). At L3-L4 there has been ossification of the disc space (arrowhead) causing ankylosis of the vertebral bodies. This appearance could be mistaken for ankylosing spondylitis except for the presence of the vacuum phenomenon at the other levels.

The ankylosis of onchronosis may be mistaken for ankylosing spondylitis. However, in ankylosing spondylitis the syndesmophytes are thin and succinct and the disc spaces are usually maintained. Examination of the sacroiliac joints on the spine film also helps to distinguish ochronosis from ankylosing spondylitis. In ochronosis the sacroiliac joints show changes of osteoarthritis, with narrowing, extensive sclerosis, and occasional vacuum phenomenon (Fig. 18–7). In ankylosing spondylitis the sacroiliac joints show erosive changes followed by ankylosis.

Generalized osteoporosis of the vertebral bodies is present, except at the end-plates, where subchondral sclerosis occurs adjacent to the degenerated discs. There is a distinct lack of osteophytes present. Their absence helps to distinguish ochronosis from other diseases that cause degenerative disc disease at multiple levels.

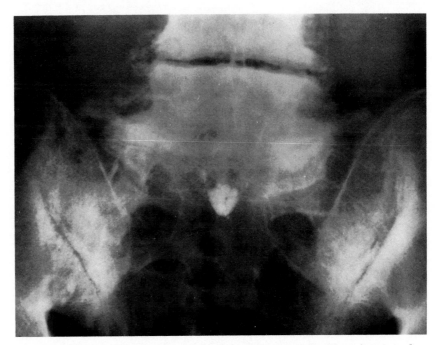

FIGURE 18–7. The sacroiliac joints in a patient with ochronosis. There is tremendous subchondral sclerosis on both sides of the sacroiliac joints bilaterally. There is a vacuum phenomenon present in both sacroiliac joints. There is no evidence of inflammatory erosion or bony ankylosis. These findings help to distinguish an ankylosed spine of ochronosis from that of ankylosing spondylitis.

The Knee

Outside of the spine the knee is the most commonly involved joint in ochronosis. Chondrocalcinosis is not part of the radiographic picture. While CPPD crystals have been identified in the synovium of the ochronotic knee, they have not been identified in the cartilage. The non-opaque ochronotic pigment deposits in the cartilage, causing degeneration. The radiographic changes are those of osteoarthritis superimposed on a uniform loss of joint space. Occasionally there is isolated lateral tibiofemoral compartment loss. The osteophytes are meager in comparison to the osteophytes seen in primary osteoarthritis (Fig. 18–8). There is a tendency toward fragmentation and the presence of multiple radiopaque intra-articular bodies. Sometimes tendinous calcification is observed.

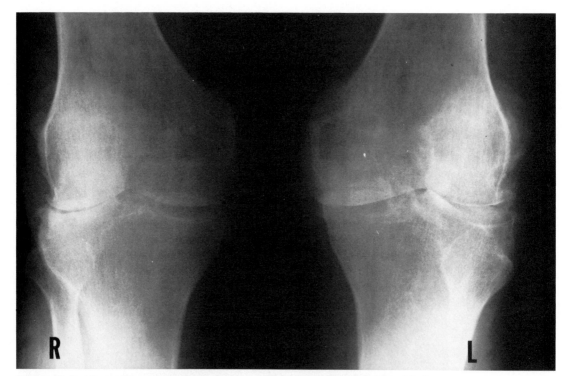

FIGURE 18–8. AP standing view of both knees in a patient with ochronosis. The right knee shows preferential lateral compartment narrowing. The left knee shows uniform narrowing. Subchondral bone sclerosis is superimposed upon the cartilage loss. There is minimal osteophyte formation considering the extensive loss of cartilage.

The Hip

The radiographic picture is that of osteoarthritis superimposed on uniform joint space narrowing. Again there is a lack of osteophytes, in contrast to the presence of osteophytes in primary osteoarthritis. In some patients severe destruction of the femoral head may be observed with multiple intra-articular bodies (Fig. 18–9). The etiology of this destruction is unknown; it has been suggested that it is secondary to osteonecrosis superimposed on the ochronotic hip.

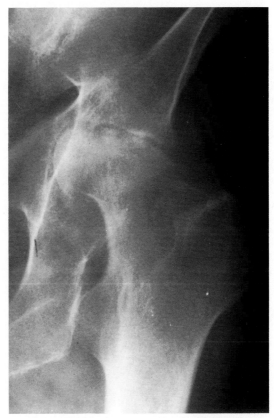

FIGURE 18–9. AP view of a hip in a patient with ochronosis. This hip demonstrates the severe destructive change that may occur in some patients with ochronosis.

The Shoulder

There is narrowing of the glenohumeral joint space with superimposed osteoarthritic changes. Fragmentation of the humeral head and tendinous calcification, if present, may help to distinguish ochronosis from osteoarthritis secondary to other deposition diseases.

SUMMARY

These three deposition diseases are relatively rare. They exhibit radiographic features of common arthropathies. However, each has distinctive features that separate it from other arthropathies. As long as the rare arthropathy is considered and the distinguishing features are observed, a correct diagnosis can be made.

SUGGESTED READINGS

Hemochromatosis

Atkins CJ, McIvor J, Smith PM, et al.: Chondrocalcinosis and arthropathy: Studies in haemochromatosis and in idiopathic chondrocalcinosis. Q J Med 39:71, 1970.
Hirsch JH, Killien C, Troupin RH: The arthropathy of hemochromatosis. Radiology 118:591, 1976.
Ross P, Wood G: Osteoarthropathy in idiopathic hemochromatosis. AJR 109:575, 1970.
Schumacher HR Jr: Hemochromatosis and arthritis. Arthritis Rheum 7:41, 1964.

Wilson's Disease

Finby N, Bearn AG: Roentgenographic abnormalities of the skeletal system in Wilson's disease (hepatolenticular degeneration). AJR 79:603, 1958.
Golding DN, Walshe JM: Arthropathy of Wilson's disease. Study of clinical and radiological features in 32 patients. Ann Rheum Dis 36:99, 1977.
Mindelzun R, Elkin M, Scheinberg IH, Sternlieb I: Skeletal changes in Wilson's disease. A radiological study. Radiology 94:127, 1970.

Ochronosis

Laskar RH, Sargison KD: Ochronotic arthropathy. A review with four case reports. J Bone Joint Surg 52B:653, 1970.
O'Brien WM, LaDu BN, Bunim JJ: Biochemical, pathologic and clinical aspects of alkaptonuria, ochronosis and ochronotic arthropathy. Am J Med 34:813, 1963.
Pagan-Carlo J, Payzant AR: Roentgenographic manifestations in a severe case of alkaptonuric osteoarthritis. AJR 80:635, 1958.
Pomeranx MM, Friedman LJ, Tunick IS: Roentgen findings in alkaptonuric ochronosis. Radiology 37:295, 1941.

chapter 19

COLLAGEN VASCULAR DISEASES (Connective Tissue Diseases)

The collagen vascular diseases (connective tissue diseases) are a group of diseases that have multiple varied systemic manifestations. Articular symptoms play a minor role in the total clinical picture and usually produce little in the way of radiographic change in the joint itself. Although each disease has distinct features, there is a tendency toward overlap among the diseases. The diseases to be discussed are systemic lupus erythematosus, scleroderma, dermatomyositis, polyarteritis nodosa, and mixed connective tissue disease (MCTD).

SYSTEMIC LUPUS ERYTHEMATOSUS (SLE)

Systemic lupus erythematosus (SLE) is the most common of the collagen vascular diseases. In this disease, articular symptoms are present in 75 to 90 per cent of patients. The radiographic changes are the following:

1. **Soft tissue swelling**

2. **Juxta-articular osteoporosis**

3. **Subluxations and dislocations**

4. Absence of erosions

5. Absence of joint space loss

6. Calcification

7. Osteonecrosis

8. Bilateral and symmetrical distribution

9. Distribution in hand and wrist, hip, knee, and shoulder

The radiographic changes divide into three different categories: (1) a deforming non-erosive arthritis, (2) osteonecrosis, and (3) calcification of soft tissue.

Deforming Non-Erosive Arthritis

A deforming non-erosive arthritis is seen most commonly in the hands and wrists (Fig. 19–1). Early in the course of the disease soft tissue swelling is seen, with eventual soft tissue atrophy. Juxta-articular osteoporosis is present which eventually becomes diffuse osteoporosis. When not distorted by subluxation or dislocation, the joint space appears preserved. Subluxation and/or dislocation without erosive disease is the hallmark of SLE. The subluxations are usually easily reducible. Therefore, deformities may not be detected on the routine PA radiograph in which the technician has carefully positioned the digits for optimum imaging. However, on the Norgaard view, in which the fingers are not positioned rigidly, the subluxations become apparent (Fig. 19–2). A similar deforming non-erosive arthritis may involve the knee or the shoulder, but it is more difficult to image radiographically.

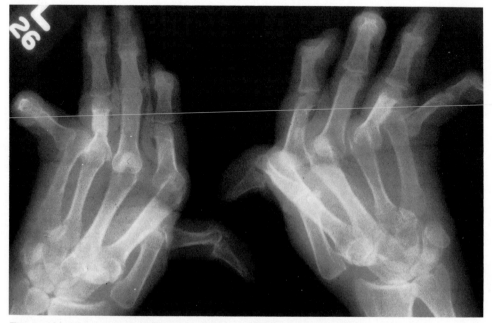

FIGURE 19–1. PA view of both hands in a patient with SLE. Osteoporosis is present. Severe subluxations of all joints are present. There is no evidence of erosive disease. This is the classic deforming non-erosive arthritis of lupus.

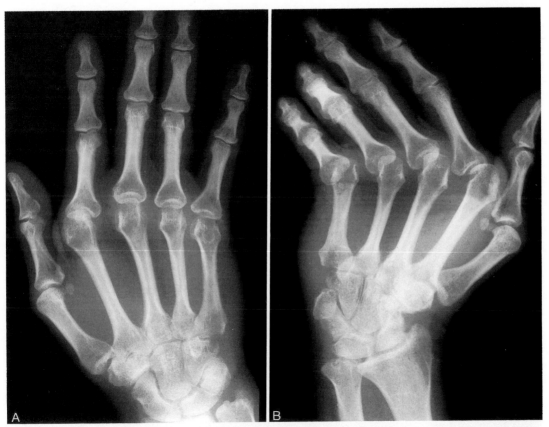

FIGURE 19–2. *A*, PA view of the hand in a patient with SLE. There is juxta-articular osteoporosis present. There is minimal subluxation of the MCP and PIP joints of the index finger. *B*, View of the same hand in the Norgaard position. The fingers have not been rigidly positioned by the technician; therefore severe subluxations of the MCP joints become apparent.

Osteonecrosis

Osteonecrosis is said to occur in 6 to 40 per cent of patients with SLE. Although most of these patients are on steroids, it is known that SLE causes osteonecrosis even in the absence of steroid treatment. The patient with SLE with a significant vasculitic component who is being treated with steroids is extremely prone to osteonecrosis. The femoral heads, the humeral heads, the femoral condyles, the tibial plateaus, and the tali are the most common sites of osteonecrosis in SLE (Fig. 19–3). However, it has also been seen in the lunates, the naviculars, and the metacarpal and metatarsal heads (Fig. 19–4). It usually occurs bilaterally and asymmetrically.

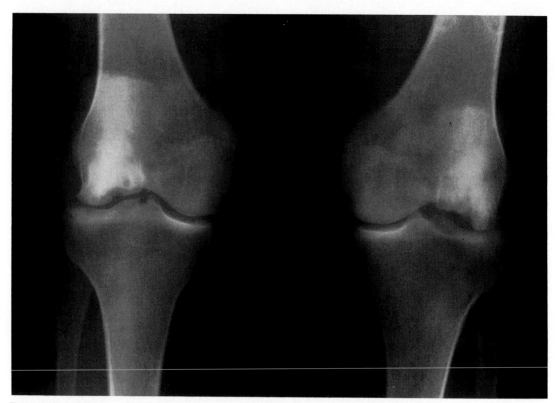

FIGURE 19–3. AP view of both knees in a patient with lupus. Osteonecrosis is observed in both lateral femoral condyles.

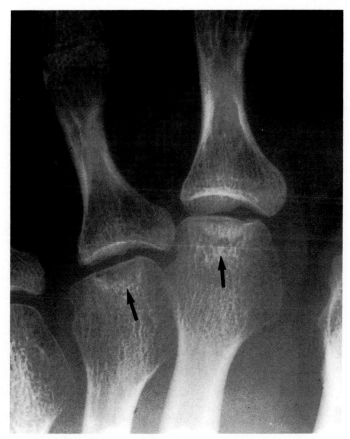

FIGURE 19–4. AP view of MTP joints in a patient with lupus. There is osteonecrosis present in the heads of the 2nd and 3rd metatarsals (arrows).

The radiographic findings are those observed in osteonecrosis of any etiology. Dead bone itself does not change radiographically. The radiographic changes observed are those of repair. The initial bone loss or osteoporosis in the repair process may not be appreciated radiographically. The first radiographic change may be increased smudgy density, which represents either dead bone that appears dense in comparison to the surrounding osteoporosis or reparative bone (Fig. 19–5). One may see a combination of osteoporosis and osteosclerosis. Advanced osteonecrosis is present when a subchondral lucency is seen (Fig. 19–6). The lucency is created by a vacuum introduced between a distracted subchondral fragment and the remaining femoral head. It represents impending collapse of the articular segment into the underlying bone, if such has not already occurred. Once the articular surface has been deformed, the actual joint undergoes secondary osteoarthritic changes.

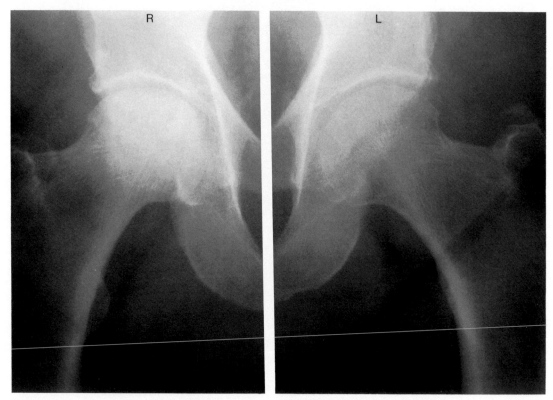

FIGURE 19–5. AP view of both hips in a patient with lupus. The left hip is normal. Increased smudgy density is observed in the right femoral head. This is an early radiographic change of osteonecrosis.

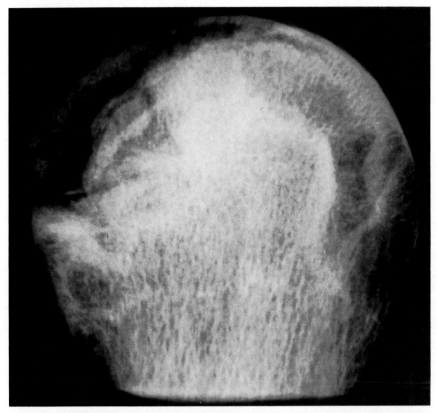

FIGURE 19–6. Specimen radiograph of a femoral head with advanced osteonecrosis. (The specimen was surgically removed from a patient with SLE.) There is a combination of osteoporosis and osteosclerosis present. A large subchondral lucency or vacuum separates the detached subchondral fragment from the underlying collapsed bone.

Calcification

Calcification may be present in the subcutaneous tissue in SLE. It is usually linear and streaky in its appearance. There is no definite association of this calcification with the deforming non-erosive arthritis or with the osteonecrosis. If seen alone, this calcification is difficult to differentiate from that of other collagen vascular diseases.

SCLERODERMA

Forty-six per cent of patients with scleroderma have articular symptoms. The radiographic changes appear to be limited to the hands and wrists. The radiographic changes are the following:

1. Resorption of soft tissue of the finger tip

2. Subcutaneous calcification

3. Erosion of the distal tuft

4. Acrosclerosis

The first visible radiographic change is the resorption of the soft tissue of the finger tip. This may or may not be accompanied by amorphous calcification (Fig. 19–7). Of the fingers involved, 40 to 80 per cent have erosion of the distal tuft. It begins on the palmar aspect of the tuft and may progress to resorb the entire distal tuft (Fig. 19–8). Rarely one may observe erosive disease of the DIP joints and/or the 1st carpometacarpal joint.

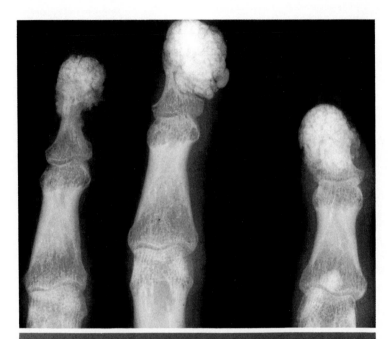

FIGURE 19–7. PA view of three digits in scleroderma. There is amorphous calcification in the soft tissues of the distal phalanges. There are accompanying erosive changes of the distal tufts.

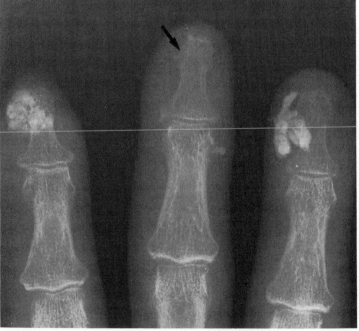

FIGURE 19–8. PA view of three digits in scleroderma. There is amorphous calcification present in the soft tissues. Early resorption of the distal tuft is seen in the middle digit (arrow).

DERMATOMYOSITIS

In patients with dermatomyositis the radiographic abnormality most commonly observed is soft tissue calcification (Fig. 19–9). This is present more often in children than in adults. It is usually identified along intermuscular fascial planes, but it may be present around joints or subcutaneously. If articular symptoms are present, there are usually no radiographic findings around the joint. Sometimes, transient osteoporosis may be seen, and there have been occasional reports of distal tuft resorption similar to that seen in scleroderma.

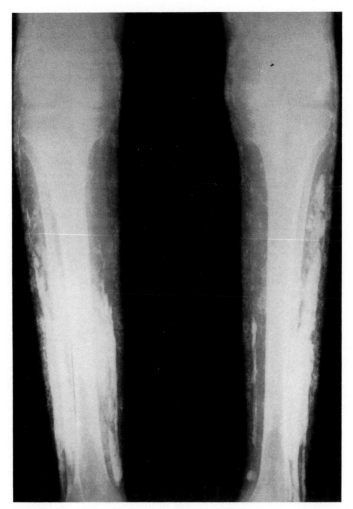

FIGURE 19–9. AP view of the lower extremities in a child with dermatomyositis. Calcification is seen along intermuscular fascial planes as well as in subcutaneous tissue.

POLYARTERITIS NODOSA

The only radiographic change reported in polyarteritis nodosa is periosteal new bone formation. This has been limited primarily to the tibia and fibula and has appeared in a symmetrical fashion.

MIXED CONNECTIVE TISSUE DISEASE (MCTD)

Mixed connective tissue disease (MCTD) was originally defined in a patient having a combination of SLE and scleroderma. Today, a patient with MCTD may have features of SLE, scleroderma, and rheumatoid arthritis. The disease entity is defined serologically. Radiographically the patient may have features of all three diseases involving primarily the hands, wrists, and feet. The radiographic features of scleroderma are soft tissue atrophy, calcification, and distal tuft resorption. Those of SLE are osteoporosis and subluxations. Those of rheumatoid arthritis are erosive disease and joint space loss. In contrast to rheumatoid arthritis, the erosive disease may include the DIP joints as well as the PIP's, MCP's, and carpal joint spaces. One should identify at least one feature of scleroderma and one feature of lupus in order to make the diagnosis radiographically (Fig. 19–10). In some patients there is a unique feature of preferential ankylosis of the capitate to the lesser multangular.

SUMMARY

Although the collagen vascular diseases have individual specific manifestations, there is a tendency to overlap among the diseases. Mixed connective tissue disease is a demonstration of this overlap; however, it is defined as a distinct entity serologically and should not be confused with the general overlap among these disease entities.

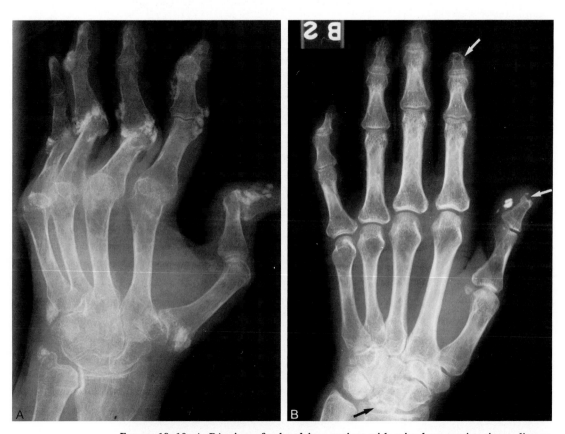

FIGURE 19–10. *A*, PA view of a hand in a patient with mixed connective tissue disease (MCTD). There is diffuse osteoporosis present with subluxations of the MCP and PIP joints. These are radiographic manifestations of SLE. There is also amorphous calcification in the soft tissues and loss of soft tissue in the distal phalanges. These are radiographic features of scleroderma. The combination is observed in MCTD. *B*, PA view of the hand in a patient with MCTD. There is osteonecrosis of the lunate (arrowhead), a radiographic feature of lupus. There is amorphous calcification in the soft tissue of the thumb and resorption of the distal tufts of the thumb and index finger (arrows). These are radiographic features of scleroderma. The combination is observed in MCTD.

SUGGESTED READINGS

Aptekar RG, Klippel JH, Becker KE, et al.: Avascular necrosis of the talus, scaphoid, and metatarsal head in systemic lupus erythematosus. Clin Orthop 101:127, 1974.

Budin JA, Feldman F: Soft tissue calcifications in systemic lupus erythematosus. AJR 124:358, 1975.

Fraser GM: The radiological manifestations of scleroderma (diffuse systemic sclerosis). Br J Dermatol 78:1, 1966.

Green N, Osmer JC: Small bone changes secondary to systemic lupus erythematosus. Radiology 90:118, 1968.

Klippel JH, Gerber LH, Pollak L, Decker JL: Avascular necroses in systemic lupus erythematosus. Silent symmetric osteonecrosis. Am J Med 67:83, 1979.

Labowitz R, Schumacher HR Jr: Articular manifestations of systemic lupus erythematosus. Ann Intern Med 74:911, 1971.

Saville PD: Polyarteritis nodosa with new bone formation. J Bone Joint Surg 38B:327, 1956.

Silver TM, Farber SJ, Bole GG, Martel W: Radiological features of mixed connective tissue disease and scleroderma–systemic lupus erythematosus overlap. Radiology 120:269, 1976.

Steiner RM, Glassman L, Schwartz MW, Vanace P: The radiological findings in dermatomyositis of childhood. Radiology 111:385, 1974.

Tuffanelli DL, Winkelmann RK: Systemic scleroderma: Clinical study of 727 cases. Arch Dermatol 84:359, 1961.

Udoff EJ, Genant HK, Kozin F, Ginsberg M: Mixed connective tissue disease: The spectrum of radiographic manifestations. Radiology 124:613, 1977.

Weissman BN, Rappoport AS, Sosman JL, Schur PH: Radiographic findings in the hands in patients with systemic lupus erythematosus. Radiology 126:313, 1978.

Yune HY, Vix VA, Klatte EC: Early fingertip changes in scleroderma. JAMA 215:1113, 1971.

chapter 20

JUVENILE CHRONIC ARTHRITIS

There are a variety of disorders that affect the joints in children. In the past all of the disorders have been lumped together and labeled juvenile rheumatoid arthritis. Although each disorder has different clinical and radiographic manifestations and course, it may be impossible to distinguish one disorder from another at a specific time within the course of the disease. Therefore, the better term "juvenile chronic arthritis" has been applied to these disorders.

Juvenile chronic arthritis (JCA) includes juvenile-onset ankylosing spondylitis, psoriatic arthritis, arthritis of inflammatory bowel disease, juvenile-onset adult type (seropositive) rheumatoid arthritis, and Still's disease (seronegative chronic arthritis). All of these disorders, except for Still's disease, tend to occur in older children and therefore usually behave like their adult counterpart. Juvenile-onset adult type (seropositive) rheumatoid arthritis differs from adult rheumatoid arthritis in two ways. First, a periostitis is frequently present in the metaphyses of the phalanges, metacarpals, and metatarsals. Second, there is significant erosive disease without joint space loss.

Still's disease (seronegative chronic arthritis) makes up 70 per cent of the cases of JCA. There are three different clinical presentations of Still's disease, with some crossover within these three groups. The three groups are (1) classic systemic disease with little to no radiographic articular changes, (2) polyarticular disease with less severe systemic manifestations, and (3) pauciarticular or monoarticular disease with infrequent systemic manifestations. Some of the children with pauciarticular or monoarticular disease progress to polyarticular disease. In all presentations the children are younger than those with other JCA. Since the articular changes are occurring in rapidly growing bones, the radiographic changes are quite different from those in the older child. The articular radiographic changes in Still's disease are as follows:

1. Periarticular soft tissue swelling

2. Osteoporosis—juxta-articular, metaphyseal lucent bands, and/or diffuse

3. Periostitis

4. Overgrown or ballooned epiphyses

5. Advanced skeletal maturation—premature fusion leading to decreased bone length

6. Late joint space loss

7. Late erosive disease

8. Ankylosis

9. Bilateral and symmetrical distribution in polyarticular disease; sporadic distribution in pauciarticular or monoarticular disease

10. Distribution in hand and wrist, foot, knee, ankle, hip, cervical spine, and mandible in decreasing order in polyarticular disease; distribution in knee, ankle, elbow, and wrist in pauciarticular or monoarticular disease

The radiographic changes are those of chronic inflammation and hyperemia in a joint that is undergoing growth and change. The changes described may occur in any juvenile chronic arthritis if the disease begins at an early enough age.

THE HAND AND WRIST

The hand is less frequently involved than the wrist. The distribution of the disease within the hand differs from that of adult RA in that the DIP joints are involved as well as the PIP and MCP joints (Fig. 20–1). In early involvement there is periarticular soft tissue swelling and juxta-articular osteoporosis. In 23 per cent a periostitis is present along the metaphyses and diaphyses of the phalanges and metacarpals. As the disease persists, there is overgrowth and ballooning of the epiphyses (Fig. 20–2). Premature fusion of the growth plate follows, leading to brachydactyly (Fig. 20–3). However, despite these changes there is usually a noticeable absence of erosive disease and the joint spaces tend to be preserved. With continuing osteoporosis, epiphyseal compression fractures develop, leading to flattening of the metacarpal heads and "cupping" of the proximal phalangeal ossification centers (Fig. 20–4). Even now growth deformity, rather than erosive disease, remains the prominent part of the radiographic picture.

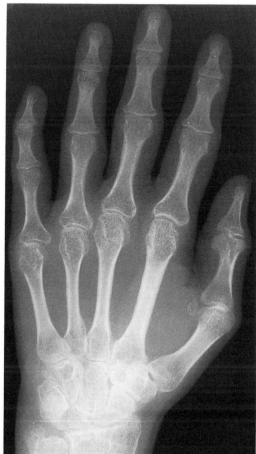

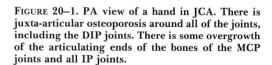

FIGURE 20–1. PA view of a hand in JCA. There is juxta-articular osteoporosis around all of the joints, including the DIP joints. There is some overgrowth of the articulating ends of the bones of the MCP joints and all IP joints.

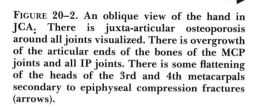

FIGURE 20–2. An oblique view of the hand in JCA. There is juxta-articular osteoporosis around all joints visualized. There is overgrowth of the articular ends of the bones of the MCP joints and all IP joints. There is some flattening of the heads of the 3rd and 4th metacarpals secondary to epiphyseal compression fractures (arrows).

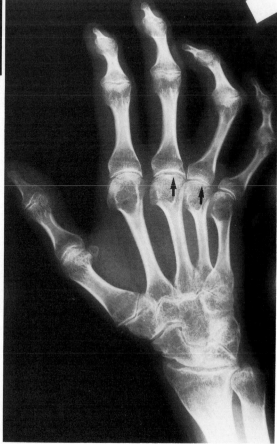

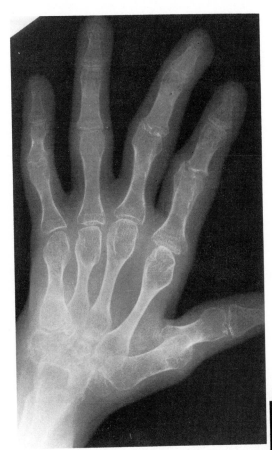

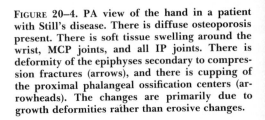

FIGURE 20–3. PA view of a hand in Still's disease. There is diffuse osteoporosis. There is marked overgrowth of the metacarpal heads with premature fusion leading to severe brachydactyly. There are erosive changes noted around the PIP joints of the index and 3rd fingers and severe destruction of the wrist.

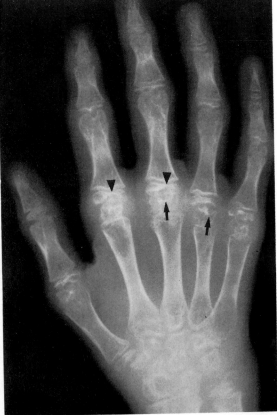

FIGURE 20–4. PA view of the hand in a patient with Still's disease. There is diffuse osteoporosis present. There is soft tissue swelling around the wrist, MCP joints, and all IP joints. There is deformity of the epiphyses secondary to compression fractures (arrows), and there is cupping of the proximal phalangeal ossification centers (arrowheads). The changes are primarily due to growth deformities rather than erosive changes.

The wrist is commonly involved. Early in the disease there is soft tissue swelling and juxta-articular osteoporosis. With persistence of the disease process, there is acceleration of growth maturation in the wrist, as seen by increase in the number and size of the carpal bones. The carpal bones become irregular in their contour secondary to erosions occurring at a young age and repairing with growth (Fig. 20–5). Nineteen per cent of patients demonstrate ankyloses at the wrist. Usually one of the three compartments of the wrist is not ankylosed. Most frequently the common carpometacarpal and midcarpal compartments are ankylosed, with total sparing of the radiocarpal compartment (Fig. 20–6).

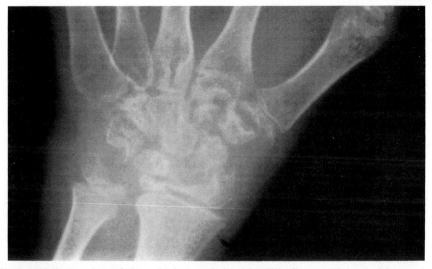

FIGURE 20–5. PA view of the wrist in a patient with Still's disease. The carpal bones are very irregular in their contour secondary to erosions occurring at a young age with subsequent repair.

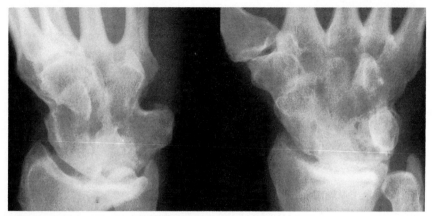

FIGURE 20–6. PA and oblique views of the wrist in a patient with Still's disease. There is ankylosis of the common carpometacarpal compartment and the midcarpal compartment. The radiocarpal compartment remains open.

THE FOOT AND ANKLE

The changes seen in the foot are similar to those seen in the hand. Initially there is soft tissue swelling and juxta-articular osteoporosis around the IP and MTP joints. Periostitis may involve the metaphyses and diaphyses of the proximal phalanges and metatarsals. Eventually there is epiphyseal overgrowth with premature fusion of the growth plate and brachydactyly (Fig. 20–7). Involvement of the tarsal bones is similar to involvement of the carpal bones. The tarsals are irregular in their shape and contour. They may be enlarged and increased in number. Bony ankylosis occurs here as it does in the carpal bones (Fig. 20–8). In the ankle there may be a tibiotalar tilt secondary to overgrowth of the epiphysis and premature closure of the epiphyseal plate (Fig. 20–9).

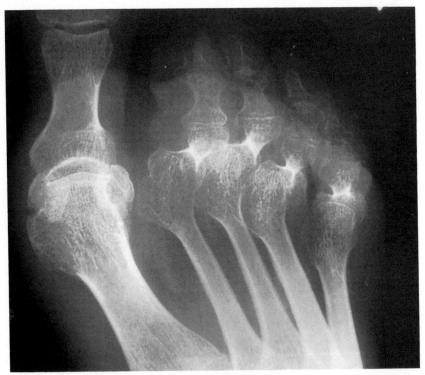

FIGURE 20–7. AP view of the foot in early Still's disease. There is osteoporosis seen in the metatarsal heads. The metatarsal heads are overgrown. There are subluxations of the MTP joints.

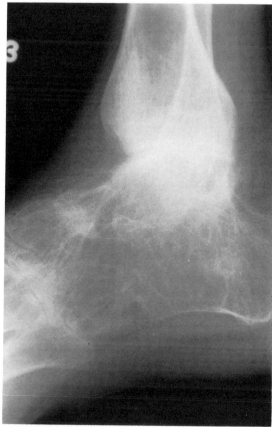

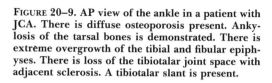

FIGURE 20–8. A lateral view of the ankle in a patient with JCA demonstrates ankylosis of the tarsal joints except at the tarsometatarsal compartment. There is also overgrowth of the articulating end of the tibia.

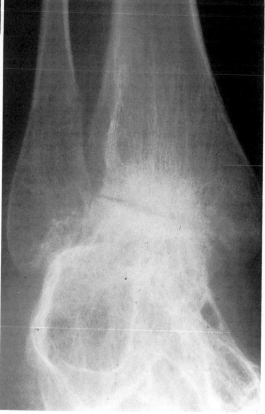

FIGURE 20–9. AP view of the ankle in a patient with JCA. There is diffuse osteoporosis present. Ankylosis of the tarsal bones is demonstrated. There is extreme overgrowth of the tibial and fibular epiphyses. There is loss of the tibiotalar joint space with adjacent sclerosis. A tibiotalar slant is present.

THE KNEE

The knee is the joint most commonly affected in pauciarticular or monoarticular disease, and it is very frequently involved in polyarticular disease. Early in the course of the disease soft tissue swelling and juxta-articular osteoporosis are present. In the knee, a metaphyseal lucent band, similar to that seen in leukemia, may be observed as a manifestation of juxta-articular osteoporosis. This is thought to be secondary to increased metaphyseal bone blood flow in the child, which accompanies increased blood flow to the inflamed synovium. Persistent hyperemia in and around the joint causes overgrowth of the femoral and tibial epiphyses (Fig. 20–10). There is widening of the intracondylar notch secondary to overgrowth of the femoral condyles. There is overgrowth of the patella with either elongation or squaring of its configuration. The radiographic changes in the knee are similar to those seen in hemophilia. Some authors have described the overgrown patella in hemophilia as more squared in appearance than in JCA. There also tend to be more cysts in the hemophilic knee secondary to intraosseous bleeding. With persistent osteoporosis there are epiphyseal compression fractures, causing a flattened appearance of the femoral condyles. In severe involvement of the knee there may be joint space narrowing and osseous erosions (Fig. 20–11).

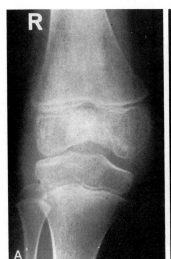
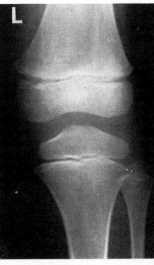
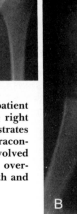
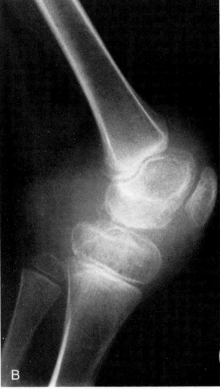

FIGURE 20–10. *A*, AP standing view of both knees in a patient with monarticular disease. The left knee is normal. The right knee, although held in a somewhat flexed position, demonstrates overgrowth of the femoral and tibial epiphyses. The intracondylar notch appears widened. *B*, Lateral view of the involved knee showing a large synovial effusion. Again there is overgrowth of the epiphyses. In addition, there are overgrowth and elongation of the patella.

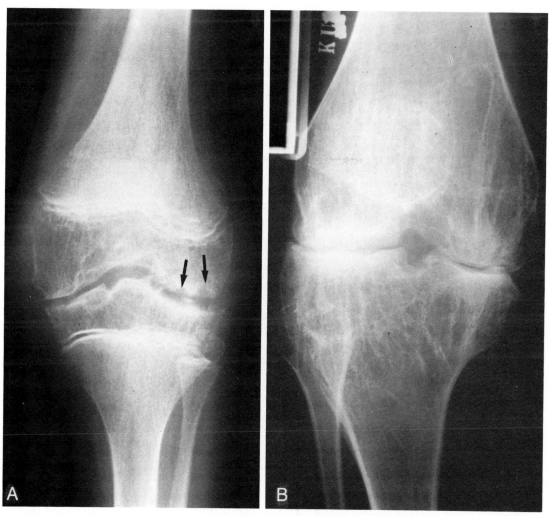

FIGURE 20–11. *A*, AP view of a knee in a patient with Still's disease. Soft tissue swelling is seen around the knee. There is overgrowth of the epiphyses and widening of the intracondylar notch. The joint space has become somewhat narrowed. The femoral condyles have become flattened. Osseous erosions are observed (arrows). *B*, AP view of the knee in an adult who had JCA. There is overgrowth of the articulating ends of the bones, indicating previous overgrowth of the epiphyses and premature fusion. There is total loss of the joint space. There are flattening of the condyles and widening of the notch. There are superimposed osteoarthritic changes present.

THE HIP

The hip is less frequently involved in Still's disease; however, it is commonly involved in the other juvenile chronic arthropathies. Again, the early change is juxta-articular osteoporosis. With time there is enlargement of the femoral epiphysis, with premature fusion of the growth plate (Fig. 20–12). The femoral head may become irregular in its outline secondary to compression fractures and erosive changes (Fig. 20–13). In advanced disease uniform joint space loss occurs with resultant protrusion of the acetabulum. Erosive changes become prominent (Fig. 20–14). In the very young patient involvement of the hip may be accompanied by hypoplasia of the ilium and a coxa valga deformity of the proximal femur.

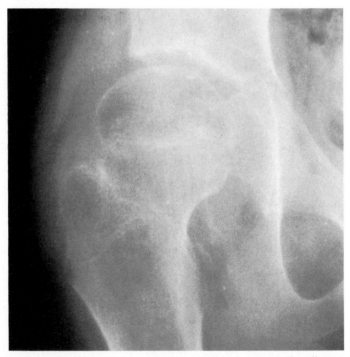

FIGURE 20–12. AP view of the hip in a patient with early monarticular disease. There is severe osteoporosis of the bony structures. The femoral head is enlarged, with its lateral margin extending beyond the articulating acetabular surface. There is evidence of beginning fusion of the epiphyseal plate which is premature for this patient.

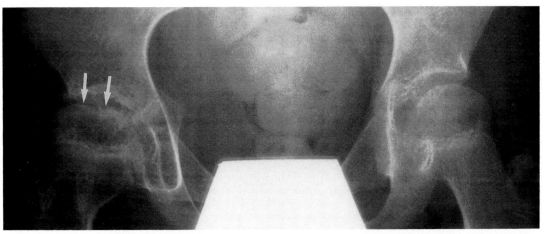

FIGURE 20–13. An AP view of the pelvis in a patient with polyarticular Still's disease. While both hips are involved, the right is more severely involved than the left. The right hip is more osteoporotic. The femoral head is irregular in its outline secondary to compression fractures (arrows).

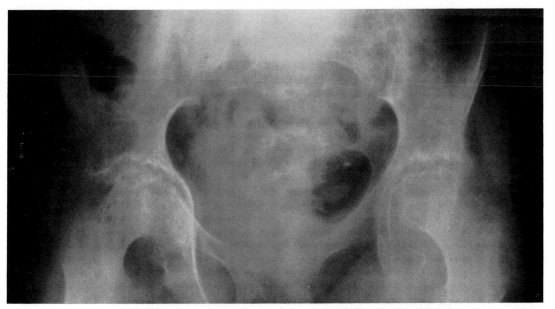

FIGURE 20–14. AP view of the pelvis in advanced disease of the hip joints. Erosive disease is present in both hips. Protrusion of the acetabulum has occurred on the right side. There is some atrophy of the left ilium.

THE CERVICAL SPINE

Atlanto-axial subluxation and/or odontoid erosion, as seen in adult RA, is common in juvenile-onset adult type (seropositive) rheumatoid arthritis but is uncommon in Still's disease. In Still's disease, the apophyseal joints are involved with ankylosis beginning in the upper cervical spine. The apophyseal joint of C2-C3 is the most commonly ankylosed. The lower cervical spine is rarely involved and never without involvement of the upper cervical spine. With the ankylosis of the apophyseal joints there is decrease in the size of the adjoining vertebral bodies and decrease in the disc space (Fig. 20–15). This decrease in size of the vertebral bodies is believed to be secondary to the ankylosis of the apophyseal joints occurring at a very young age. It is not seen in juvenile-onset ankylosing spondylitis, when the ankylosis of the apophyseal joints occurs at a much older age.

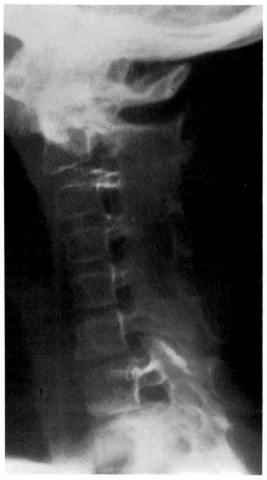

FIGURE 20–15. Lateral view of the neck in a child with Still's disease. There is total ankylosis of the apophyseal joints from C2 through C6. The apophyseal joint of C6-C7 remains open. Hypoplasia of the C3, C4, and C5 vertebral bodies is present. This hypoplasia is believed to be secondary to the ankylosis of the apophyseal joints occurring at a very young age.

THE MANDIBLE

Ten to 20 per cent of the children with Still's disease have underdevelopment of the mandible. There is shortening of the body and the vertical rami of the mandible. A concavity develops on the undersurface of the mandible. The condyles of the mandible are flattened and poorly developed. This may or may not lead to temporomandibular joint changes.

SUMMARY

The radiographic changes of juvenile chronic arthritis depend upon the age of onset of the specific disease. If the disease begins in the older child, the radiographic findings mimic the similar adult arthropathy. If the disease onset is in the young child, growth disturbances, rather than joint space loss and erosion, become the predominant picture.

SUGGESTED READINGS

Ansell BM: Chronic arthritis in childhood. Ann Rheum Dis 37:107, 1978.

Ansell BM, Kent PA: Radiological changes in juvenile chronic polyarthritis. Skel Radiol 1:129, 1977.

Becker MH, Coccaro PJ, Converse JM: Antegonial notching of mandible: An often overlooked mandibular deformity in congenital and acquired disorders. Radiology 121:149, 1976.

Chaplin D, Pulkki T, Saarimaa A, Vainio K: Wrist and finger deformities in juvenile rheumatoid arthritis. Acta Rheum Scand 15:206, 1969.

Jacqueline F, Boujot A, Canet L: Involvement of hips in juvenile rheumatoid arthritis. Arthritis Rheum 4:500, 1961.

Martel W, Holt JF, Cassidy JT: Roentgenologic manifestations of juvenile rheumatoid arthritis. AJR 88:400, 1962.

Sairanen E: On rheumatoid arthritis in children: Clinicoroentgenological study. Acta Rheum Scand Suppl 2:1, 1958.

chapter 21

HEMOPHILIA

The joint changes in hemophilia are secondary to chronic repetitive hemarthrosis and intraosseous bleeding. Hemarthrosis occurs in 75 to 90 per cent of patients with hemophilia. The first bleed usually occurs between the ages of two and three. Repetitive bleeding episodes occur between the ages of eight and thirteen, with 50 per cent of patients developing permanent bone changes around the joint. The radiographic change in the joint depends upon the age of the patient at the time of the bleed, the site of the bleed, and the acuteness or chronicity of the bleed. The articular changes in hemophilia are the following:

1. **Radiodense soft tissue swelling**

2. **Osteoporosis—juxta-articular or diffuse**

3. **Overgrown or ballooned epiphyses**

4. **Subchondral cysts**

5. **Late uniform joint space loss**

6. **Late secondary osteoarthritic changes**

7. **Asymmetrical sporadic distribution**

8. **Distribution in knee, elbow, ankle, hip, and shoulder in decreasing order. Changes distal to the elbow or ankle are rare.**

Radiographic changes of hemophilia resemble those of juvenile chronic arthritis except that there are usually no inhibition of growth, no periostitis, and no bone ankylosis.

THE KNEE

The knee is the joint most commonly involved in hemophilia. In the acute hemarthrosis, joint effusion and juxta-articular osteoporosis are observed. If chronic bleeding occurs, the joint effusion becomes radio-dense (Fig. 21–1). Chronic hyperemia to the joint leads to overgrowth or ballooning of the femoral and tibial epiphyses. The overgrowth of the femoral condyles causes widening of the intracondylar notch. This widening may be accentuated by the position of the knee, which is frequently held in fixed flexion. The condyles may appear flattened. The patella is ballooned and squared inferiorly. Multiple subchondral cysts are usually visualized in the epiphyses (Fig. 21–2). If the chronic bleeding occurs in an older child, the overgrowth of the epiphyses and widening of the intracondylar notch may not be as apparent as in the younger child (Fig. 21–3). In chronic phases of the disease there may be uniform joint space loss with secondary osteoarthritic changes (Fig. 21–4).

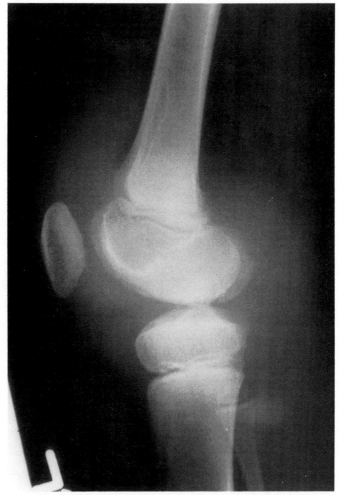

FIGURE 21–1. Lateral view of the knee in a patient with hemophilia. A radiodense effusion is present. There is overgrowth of the epiphyses, as well as ballooning of the patella.

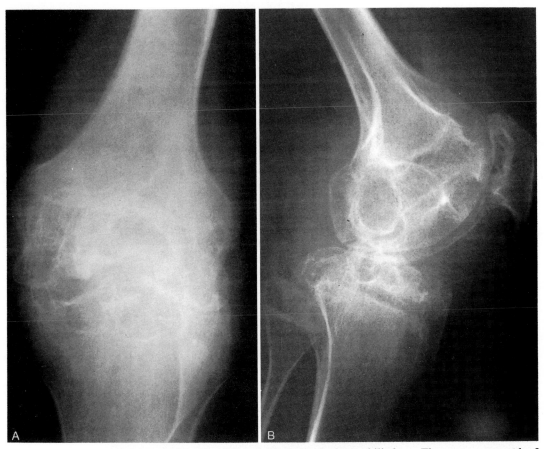

FIGURE 21–2. AP (*A*) and lateral (*B*) views of a hemophilic knee. There are overgrowth of the epiphyses, widening of the intracondylar notch, ballooning of the patella, and squaring of its inferior border. Huge subchondral cysts are present.

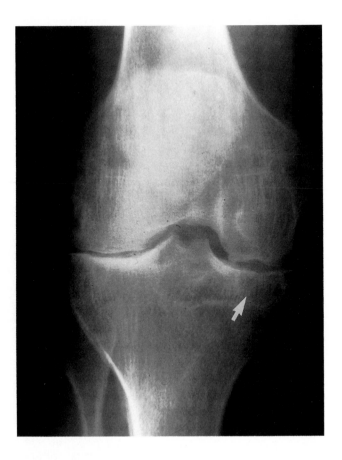

FIGURE 21–3. AP view of the knee in a 21-year-old patient with hemophilia. The overgrowth of the epiphyses and widening of the intracondylar notch are not as easily discernible as in Figure 21–2. There is uniform loss of the joint space and a subchondral cyst is present (arrow).

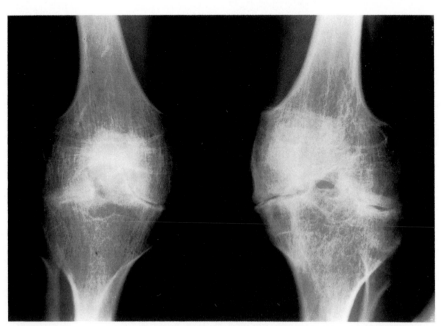

FIGURE 21–4. AP view of both knees in a patient with long-standing hemophilia. The radiographic changes are those of chronic disease. There are ballooning of the epiphyses and widening as well as deepening of the intracondylar notches. There is flattening of the femoral condyles. There are superimposed secondary osteoarthritic changes present.

THE ANKLE

Again, in the acute bleed, soft tissue swelling and juxta-articular osteoporosis are observed. The soft tissue swelling becomes radiodense in the chronic joint. There is overgrowth of the tibial epiphysis. This may be accompanied by premature fusion of the epiphyseal plate and abnormal growth or flattening of the talus. The combination leads to a tibiotalar slant (Fig. 21–5). In late involvement there may be uniform loss of the joint space with superimposed secondary osteoarthritic changes.

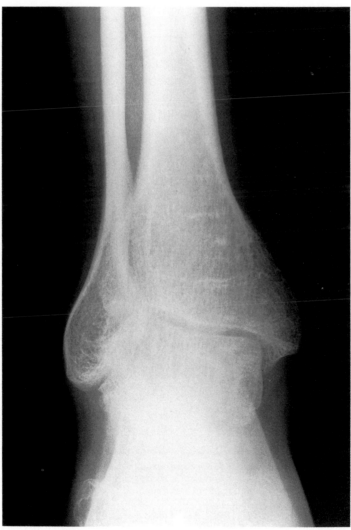

FIGURE 21–5. AP view of the ankle in a patient with long-standing hemophilia. There is ballooning of the epiphyses of the tibia and fibula. There is a tibiotalar slant indicating premature fusion of the epiphyseal plate.

THE ELBOW

Radiodense soft tissue swelling is seen around the elbow, accompanied by osteoporosis (Fig. 21–6). There may be widening of the trochlear and radial notches in the ulna. The radial head may be enlarged and flattened. Subchondral cysts may be seen. Eventually there may be uniform loss of the joint space (Fig. 21–7).

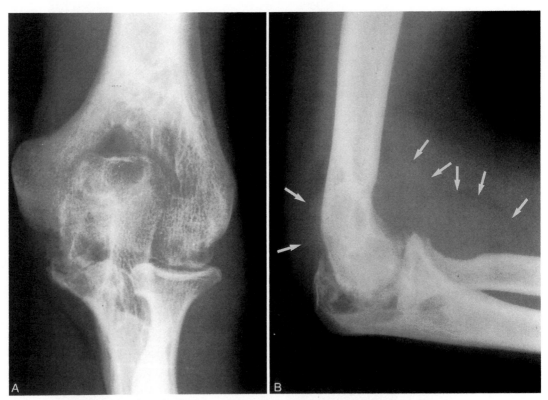

FIGURE 21–6. AP (A) and lateral (B) views of the elbow in a patient with long-standing hemophilia. Hypertrophy of the synovium is seen (arrows). There is loss or destruction of the joint space. There are enlargement and flattening of the radial head.

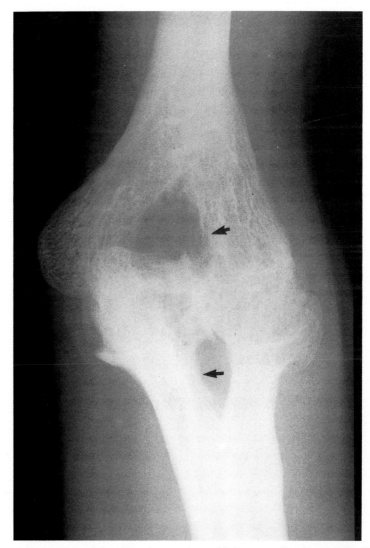

FIGURE 21–7. AP view of the elbow in a patient with long-standing hemophilia. There is overgrowth of the epiphyses. There is widening of the olecranon fossa and radial notch (arrows). There is secondary osteoarthritis present.

THE SHOULDER

Unlike the other joints described, the shoulder joint may show widening of the joint space with the hemarthrosis (Fig. 21–8). The humeral head is displaced inferiorly and laterally from its normal articulation with the glenoid. There may be radiodensity to the soft tissue around the shoulder. Overgrowth of the humeral epiphysis may be observed. Subchondral cyst formation is seen in the humeral head as well as the glenoid (Fig. 21–9). Chronic involvement may lead to uniform joint space narrowing with secondary osteoarthritic changes.

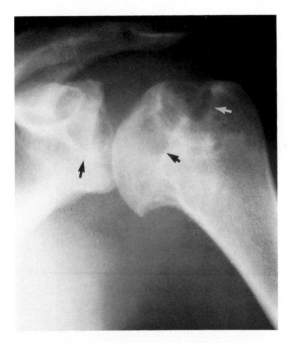

FIGURE 21–8. AP view of the shoulder in hemophilia. The joint space is widened, with the humeral head displaced inferiorly and laterally from the articulating glenoid. Subchondral cysts are present (arrows).

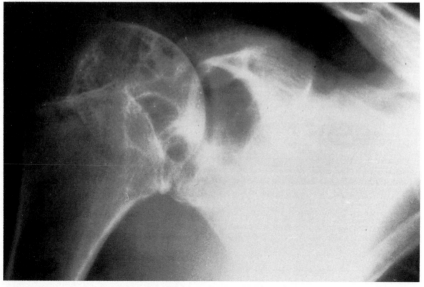

FIGURE 21–9. AP view of the shoulder in hemophilia. The joint space appears to be maintained. There is juxta-articular osteoporosis. Huge subchondral cysts are present in the humeral head as well as in the glenoid.

OTHER APPENDICULAR SITES

In the non–weight-bearing joints actual widening of the joint space may be the initial radiographic sign of an acute hemarthrosis. If the chronic hemarthrosis occurs in a small joint or in a non-growing joint, one should expect to see eventual uniform loss of joint space, with subchondral cyst formation dominating the picture (Fig. 21–10). Changes in the hip are similar to those in the shoulder, with some overgrowth of the femoral head and subchondral cyst formation. With chronic bleeding the femoral head may undergo changes of osteonecrosis.

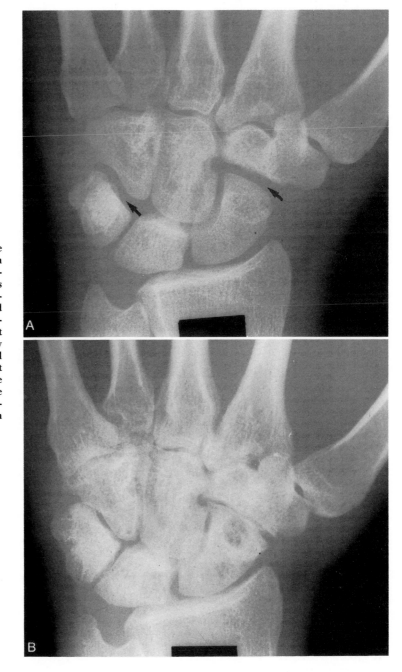

FIGURE 21–10. *A*, PA view of the wrist in a hemophiliac with acute hemorrhage. There is widening of the carpal joint spaces best identified between the navicular and multangulars and between the triquetrum and hamate (arrows). *B*, The same wrist three years later. There is now narrowing of some of the carpal joint spaces, particularly that between the navicular and the multangulars. There is a large cyst in the articulating navicular. There are cystic changes in the other carpal bones as well.

PSEUDOTUMORS

Although the radiographic changes in hemophilia most frequently occur around the joint, changes may occur at a distance from the joint. Chronic repetitive bleeding into the bone, subperiosteally, or into the soft tissue presents as a mass called a "pseudotumor." The radiographic appearance depends upon the location and extent of the bleed. The intraosseous pseudotumor may be small or large and centrally or eccentrically located. It is usually a radiolucent lesion with a well-defined border that may or may not be sclerotic. It is often septated. There may be cortical destruction with varying degrees of periosteal bone formation. The most common sites are the femur, the pelvis, and the tibia in decreasing order (Fig. 21–11). If the bleed is subperiosteal, there may be scalloping of the underlying cortex as well as profound periosteal bone formation (Fig. 21–12). The periostitis may simulate that seen with malignancy. Knowledge of the patient's underlying disease should exclude this latter possibility. A soft tissue pseudotumor may cause pressure erosion on any adjacent bone.

SUMMARY

The bone changes in hemophilia divide into (1) those associated with bleeding into the joint and (2) those associated with bleeding into or adjacent to bone away from the joint. The arthropathy may mimic that of juvenile chronic arthritis. However, presence of radiodense soft tissue swelling and subchondral cysts should help to distinguish hemophilia from juvenile chronic arthritis. Radiographically pseudotumors mimic a variety of true tumors. However, knowledge of the patient's underlying disorder should prevent misdiagnosis.

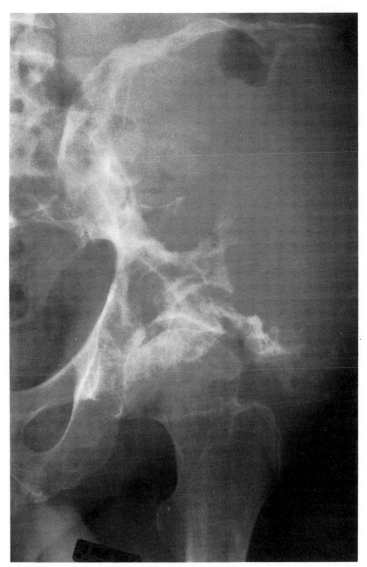

FIGURE 21–11. Huge pseudotumor involving the entire left ilium of a patient with hemophilia.

→

FIGURE 21–12. Evolution of a pseudotumor of hemophilia. *A*, PA view of the wrist in October, 1962, showing a Salter II fracture of the distal radius and a torus fracture of the distal ulna (arrow). *B*, PA view of the same wrist in June, 1963. Tremendous soft tissue swelling is present around the distal forearm. There is a bowing deformity of the distal end of the ulna. There is a large cystic septated lesion involving the distal diametaphyseal area of the radius. The cortex has been disrupted in places. There is solid periosteal response proximal to this lesion. *C*, PA view of the same wrist in August, 1964. Patient received radiation therapy in the interval. There remains some soft tissue swelling around the distal ulna. The cystic septated lesion in the distal radius has become well corticated and well defined. *D*, PA view of the same wrist and distal radius and ulna in December, 1970. The patient has continued to bleed into the forearm. In addition to the cystic septated lesion involving the distal end of the radius, there is now a large soft tissue mass with a spiculated periosteal reaction surrounding the distal end of the radius. This indicates not only intraosseous bleeding, but also subperiosteal bleeding, forming a huge pseudotumor.

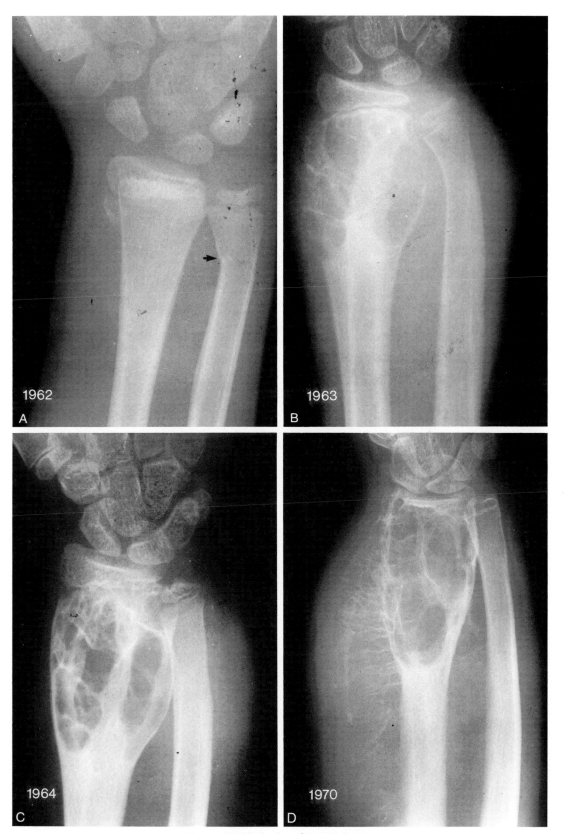

1962
A

1963
B

1964
C

1970
D

FIGURE 21–12. *See legend on opposite page*

SUGGESTED READINGS

Brant EE, Jordan HH: Radiologic aspects of hemophilic pseudotumors in bone. AJR 115:525, 1972.

Gilbert M, Cockin J: An evaluation of the radiological changes in haemophilic arthropathy of the knee. *In* Ala F, Denson KWE (eds.): Proceedings of the 7th Congress of the World Federation of Haemophilia. Amsterdam, Excerpta Medica, 1973, p 191.

Handelsman JE: The knee joint in hemophilia. Orthop Clin North Am 10:139, 1979.

Jensen PS, Putman CE: Hemophilic pseudotumor. Diagnosis, treatment and complications. Am J Dis Child 129:717, 1975.

Johnson JB, Davis TW, Bullock WH: Bone and joint changes in hemophilia. Radiology 63:64, 1954.

Jordan HH: Hemophilic Arthropathies. Springfield, IL, Charles C Thomas, Publisher 1958.

Newcomer NB: The joint changes in hemophilia. Radiology 32:573, 1939.

Pettersson H, Ahlberg A, Nilsson IM: A radiologic classification of hemophilic arthropathy. Clin Orthop Rel Res 149:153, 1980.

Stoker DJ, Murray RO: Skeletal changes in hemophilia and other bleeding disorders. Semin Roentgenol 9(3):185–193, 1974.

Zimbler S, McVerry B, Levine P: Hemophilic arthropathy of the foot and ankle. Orthop Clin North Am 7:985, 1976.

INDEX

Page numbers in *italics* indicate illustrations.